Opto-VLSI Devices and Circuits for Biomedical and Healthcare Applications

The text comprehensively discusses the latest Opto-VLSI devices and circuits useful for healthcare and biomedical applications. It further emphasizes the importance of smart technologies such as artificial intelligence, machine learning, and the internet of things for the biomedical and healthcare industries.

- Discusses advanced concepts in the field of electro-optics devices for medical applications.
- Presents optimization techniques including logical effort, particle swarm optimization and genetic algorithm to design Opto-VLSI devices and circuits.
- Showcases the concepts of artificial intelligence and machine learning for smart medical devices and data auto-collection for distance treatment.
- Covers advanced Opto-VLSI devices including a field-effect transistor and optical sensors, spintronic and photonic devices.
- Highlights application of flexible electronics in health monitoring and artificial intelligence integration for better medical devices.

The text presents the advances in the fields of optics and VLSI and their applicability in diverse areas including biomedical engineering and the healthcare sector. It covers important topics such as FET biosensors, optical biosensors and advanced optical materials. It further showcases the significance of smart technologies such as artificial intelligence, machine learning and the internet of things for the biomedical and healthcare industries. It will serve as an ideal design book for senior undergraduate, graduate students, and academic researchers in the fields including electrical engineering, electronics and communication engineering, computer engineering and biomedical engineering.

Opto-VLSI Devices and Circuits for Biomedical and Healthcare Applications

Edited by
Ankur Kumar
Sajal Agarwal
Vikrant Varshney
Varun Mishra
Yogesh Kumar Verma
Suman Lata Tripathi

CRC CRC Press
Taylor & Francis Group
Boca Raton London New York

CRC Press is an imprint of the
Taylor & Francis Group, an **informa** business

Front cover image: Andrey Suslov/Shutterstock

First edition published 2024
by CRC Press
2385 NW Executive Center Dr, Suite 320, Boca Raton, FL 33431

and by CRC Press
4 Park Square, Milton Park, Abingdon, Oxon, OX14 4RN

CRC Press is an imprint of Taylor & Francis Group, LLC

ISBN: 978-1-032-39283-7 (hbk)
ISBN: 978-1-032-55525-6 (pbk)
ISBN: 978-1-003-43113-8 (ebk)

DOI: 10.1201/9781003431138

Typeset in Sabon
by SPi Technologies India Pvt Ltd (Straive)

Contents

Notes on the Editors

Dr Ankur Kumar is an assistant professor in the school of electronics at the Indian Institute of Information Technology, Una, Himachal Pradesh. He received his PhD degree from the department of electronics and communication engineering, Motilal Nehru National Institute of Technology, Allahabad, India in October 2020. He received his MTech degree in microelectronics and VLSI design from Motilal Nehru National Institute of Technology Allahabad, India in 2016. He received his BTech degree in electronics and communication engineering from Uttar Pradesh Technical University, Lucknow, India in 2014. He contributed more than 20 research papers to various international book chapters, conferences and journals during his PhD, and one research paper during his MTech. He has participated in the organization of various conferences, summer training programs, workshops and courses coordinated by the department of electronics and communication engineering, at Motilal Nehru National Institute of Technology, Allahabad. As a member of the organizing committee he assisted with various conferences, FDPs, and webinars in electronics and communication engineering, at Meerut Institute of Engineering and Technology, Meerut. He is also peer reviewer of various international journals like *JCSC*, *Integration: the VLSI journal* and *Analog Circuits and Signal Processing* among others. He is the student chair of the solid-state devices chapter of the student branch. He has also been an active professional member of the IEEE organization since 2016. His current research interests focus on low-power VLSI circuit design and high-speed low power analog/mixed-signal processing circuits.

Dr Sajal Agarwal is currently working as assistant professor, in the department of electronics engineering, Rajiv Gandhi Institute of Petroleum Technology, Jais. She has worked at Jaypee Institute of Information Technology Noida in the electronics and communication engineering department for two years. She has more than five years of experience in academia. Her areas of research interest include optical devices, nanodevices, device fabrication, and advanced engineered materials among others. She has had several papers and book chapters published in journals, books and conferences of repute. She has served as reviewer in various international and peer-reviewed journals and conferences. She has also worked as convener and session chair for a range of international conferences, and has organized various faculty development programs and workshops. She has guided several BTech projects. She is an active member of IEEE and faculty advisor of IEEE student branch at Rajiv Gandhi Institute of Petroleum Technology, Jais.

Dr Vikrant Varshney has been working as applications engineer, Sr I in Synopsys India Pvt. Ltd., India since November 2022. Previously, he was assistant professor in the department of electronics and communication engineering, Meerut Institute of Engineering and Technology, Meerut, India from October 2020 to October 2022. He received his MTech degree in microelectronics and VLSI design and his PhD degree in electronics and communication engineering from Motilal Nehru National Institute of Technology, Allahabad, Prayagraj, India in 2015 and 2020, respectively. He received his BTech degree in electronics and communication engineering from Gautam Buddha Technical University, Lucknow, India in 2013. He has had more than 20 research papers published in referred IEEE, Springer, Elsevier and World Scientific international journals and conferences. He has also contributed more than five book chapters for various international Scopus indexed Springer and CRC book series. He has received two best paper awards at IEEE UPCON-2018 and CICT-2019. He has helped to organize and volunteered at international conferences including VCAS-2018, VCAS-2019 and VCAS-2020. He has arranged several FDPs, workshops, summer internships and expert lectures for students. He is also peer reviewer of various international journals like *JCSC* and *Silicon*. He has also been an active professional member of the IEEE organization since 2016 and has been involved in different professional activities along with academic work. He was a member of the pre-university programs sub-committee at IEEE UP Section, India. He is counselor with the IEEE student branch at MIET Meerut. His research areas of expertise include high-speed VLSI devices, VLSI device modeling and characterization, low-voltage high-speed VLSI circuit design in the area of analog/mixed-signal systems, and noise and variance-tolerant domino circuits for low-power applications.

Dr Varun Mishra received his PhD in microelectronics and VLSI from MNNIT, Allahabad. He received his MTech in VLSI design from Uttarakhand Technical University, Dehradun and BTech in electronics and communication engineering from Graphic Era University, Dehradun. He is associated with Graphic Era (deemed to be a university) as an assistant professor with more than three years of experience in academia. He has had more than 19 research papers published in SCI indexed journals and more than 19 research papers in international conference proceedings. His areas of expertise include modeling and simulation of novel semiconductor devices such as tunnel FETs, negative capacitance FETs, HEMTs, and so on, and low-power VLSI circuit design. He has served as reviewer in various International and peer reviewed Journals like Silicon, Semiconductor Science and Technology,

IJNM and conferences. He has guided several M Tech Dissertations and B Tech projects. He has given guest lectures at several institutes and organized FDPs, TDPs, and workshops. He is also an active professional member of IEEE organization.

Dr Yogesh Kumar Verma received his PhD in microelectronics and VLSI from MNNIT, Allahabad. He completed his MTech in digital systems at Uttar Pradesh Technical University, Lucknow, Uttar Pradesh, India and his BTech in electronics and communication engineering from Hindustan College of Science and Technology, Mathura, Uttar Pradesh, India. He is presently working as assistant professor with more than three years of experience in academia at Lovely Professional University, Jalandhar, Punjab, India. He has had research papers published in SCI indexed journals and international conference proceedings. His areas of expertise include modeling and simulation of novel semiconductor devices such as HEMTs and tunnel FETs. He has served as reviewer in various international and peer-reviewed journals. He has guided several BTech projects and is presently supervising PhD students.

Dr Suman Lata Tripathi received her PhD in the area of microelectronics and VLSI from MNNIT, Allahabad. She did her MTech in electronics engineering at UP Technical University, Lucknow and her BTech in electrical engineering at Purvanchal University, Jaunpur. She is associated with Lovely Professional University as a professor, with more than seventeen years of experience in academia. She has had more than 55 research papers published in referred IEEE, Springer and IOP science journals and conferences. She has also had nine Indian patents and one copyright published. She has organized several workshops, summer internships and expert lectures for students. She has worked as a session chair, conference steering committee member, editorial board member and reviewer in international/national IEEE journals and conferences. She received the Research Excellence Award in 2019 at Lovely Professional University. She also received the best paper at IEEE ICICS-2018. She has edited more than 12 books and one book series in different areas of electronics and electrical engineering. She is associated for editing work with top publishers like Elsevier, CRC Taylor & Francis, Wiley-IEEE, SP Wiley, Nova Science and Apple Academic Press among others. She has had edited books published, titled *Recent Advancement in Electronic Device, Circuit and Materials* by Nova science publishers, *Advanced VLSI Design and Testability Issues* and *Electronic Devices and Circuit Design Challenges for IoT application* by CRC Taylor & Francis and Apple Academic Press. She is also associated as an editor of a book Series on *Green Energy: Fundamentals, Concepts, and Applications* and *Design and Development of Energy efficient systems* to be published by Scrivener Publishing, Wiley (in production). She is also associated with Wiley-IEEE for her multi-authored (ongoing) book in the area of VLSI design with HDLs. She is also working as series editor for the title, *Smart Engineering Systems*, with CRC, Taylor & Francis. She has already completed one book with Elsevier on *Electronic Device and Circuits Design Challenges to Implement Biomedical Applications*. She is guest editor of a special issue in *Current Medical Imaging*, Bentham Science. She is associated as senior member IEEE, Fellow IETE and life member ISC and is always involved in different professional activities along with academic work. Her areas of expertise include microelectronics device modeling and characterization, low-power VLSI circuit design, VLSI design of testing, and advance FET design for IoT, embedded system design and biomedical applications among others.

Contributors

Manoj Singh Adhikari
School of Electronics and Electrical
  Engineering
Lovely Professional University,
  Jalandhar, Punjab, India

Sajal Agarwal
Department of Electronics
  Engineering
Rajiv Gandhi Institute of Petroleum
  Technology, Jais, India

Geetanjali Balutia
Department of Electronics and
  Communication Engineering
THDC Institute of Hydropower
  Engineering and Technology,
  Tehri, Uttarakhand, India

Chetna Bisht
Department of Electronics and
  Communication Engineering
Graphic Era (deemed to be a
  university), Uttarakhand, India

Bhartendu Chaturvedi
Department of Electronics and
  Communication Engineering
Jaypee Institute of Information
  Technology, Noida, Uttar
  Pradesh, India

R. K. Chauhan
Department of Electronics and
  Communication Engineering
Madan Mohan Malaviya University
  of Technology, Gorakhpur,
  Uttar Pradesh, India

Abhinav Gupta
Department of Applied Science and
  Humanities
Rajkiya Engineering College
  Sonbhadra, Sonbhadra,
  Uttar Pradesh, India

Akanksha Gupta
United Institute of Pharmacy,
  Prayagraj, Uttar Pradesh,
  India

Tarun Kumar Gupta
Department of Electronics and
  Communication Engineering
Maulana Azad National Institute of
  Technology Bhopal,
  Uttar Pradesh, India

Jitender
Department of Electronics and
  Communication Engineering
Ajay Kumar Garg Engineering
  College, Ghaziabad, India

Shruti Kalra
Department of Electronics
  and Communication
  Engineering
Jaypee Institute of Information
  Technology, Noida,
  Uttar Pradesh, India

Jyoti Kandpal
Department of Electronics and
  Communication Engineering
Graphic Era (deemed to be a
  university), Uttarakhand,
  India

Kavindra Kumar Kavi
Department of Electronics and
  Communication Engineering
Motilal Nehru National Institute of
  Technology Allahabad,
  Uttar Pradesh, India

Saurabh Kumar
Department of Electronics and
  Communication Engineering
Madan Mohan Malaviya University
  of Technology, Gorakhpur,
  Uttar Pradesh, India

Shailendra Kumar
Indian Space Research
  Organization, Headquarters,
  Bangalore, India

Vinay Kumar
Department of Electronics and
  Communication Engineering
Graphic Era (deemed to be a
  university), Uttarakhand,
  India

R. A. Mishra
Department of Electronics and
  Communication Engineering
Motilal Nehru National Institute of
  Technology Allahabad,
  Uttar Pradesh, India

Varun Mishra
Department of Electronics and
  Communication Engineering
Graphic Era (deemed to be a
  university), Uttarakhand, India

Vimal Kumar Mishra
Department of Electronics and
  Communication Engineering
Jaypee Institute of Information
  Technology, Noida,
  Uttar Pradesh, India

Jitendra Mohan
Department of Electronics and
  Communication Engineering
Jaypee Institute of Information
  Technology, Noida,
  Uttar Pradesh, India

Rajendra Kumar Nagaria
Department of Electronics and
  Communication Engineering
Motilal Nehru National Institute of
  Technology Allahabad, India

Amit Kumar Pandey
Department of Applied Science and
  Humanities
Rajkiya Engineering College,
  Uttar Pradesh, India

Vikas Patel
Department of Applied Science and
  Humanities
Rajkiya Engineering College,
  Uttar Pradesh, India

Praful Ranjan
Government Girls Polytechnic,
  Varanasi, India

Anurag Sewak
Department of Applied Science and
  Humanities
Rajkiya Engineering College
  Sonbhadra, Sonbhadra,
  Uttar Pradesh, India

Karan Singh
Department of Electronics and
Communication Engineering
Jaypee Institute of Information
Technology, Noida,
Uttar Pradesh, India

Priyanka Singh
Department of Electronics and
Communication Engineering
Motilal Nehru National Institute of
Technology Allahabad, India

Srishti
Department of Electronics and
Communication Engineering
Graphic Era (deemed to be a
university), Uttarakhand, India

Akash Srivastava
Department of Physics and
Electronics
KNIPSS Sultanpur, Uttar Pradesh,
India

Shivangi Srivastava
Department of Electronics
Engineering
Rajiv Gandhi Institute of Petroleum
Technology, Jais, India

Chandni Tiwari
Department of Electronics and
Communication Engineering
Graphic Era (deemed to be a
university), Uttarakhand, India

Vikas Tiwari
Department of Electronics
and Communication
Engineering
Motilal Nehru National Institute
of Technology, Allahabad,
India

Shipra Upadhyay
Department of Electrical and
Electronics Engineering
Atria Institute of Technology,
Karnataka, India

Vikrant Varshney
Electronic Design Automation
Group (EDAG), Circuit
Design & TCAD Solutions,
Synopsys (India) Pvt. Ltd.,
India

Yogesh Kumar Verma
School of Electronics and Electrical
Engineering
Lovely Professional University,
Jalandhar, Punjab, India

Nagalakshmi Yarlagadda
School of Electronics and Electrical
Engineering
Lovely Professional University,
Jalandhar, Punjab, India

Abbreviations

ABB	Active Building Block
AI	Artificial Intelligence
AMS	Analog and Mixed-Signal
AN	Artificial Network
ANN	Artificial Neural Networks
AP	All Pass
APF	All Pass Filter
BBT	Band to Band Tunneling
BGN	Band Gap Narrowing
BJT	Bipolar Junction Transistor
BOD	Biochemical Oxygen Emand
BP	Band Pass
BPNN	Backpropagation Neural Network
BR	Band Reject
BRE	Bio Recognition Element
CAD	Computer Aided Design
CB	ChubbyBrain
CBR	Case-Based Reasoning
CC	Current Conveyor
CDC	Centers for Disease Control and Prevention
CFM	Carbon Fiber Microelectrode
CGM	Continuous Glucose Monitoring
CM	Current Mode
CMOS	Complementary Metal-Oxide-Semiconductor
CMOS	Complementary MOSFET
CNN	Convolutional Neural Networks
CNTs	Carbon Nanotubes
CoV	Coronavirus
COVID-19	Coronavirus Disease 2019
CPU	Central Processing Unit
CT	Computed Tomography
CVD	Chemical Vapor Deposition
DARPA	Defense Advanced Research Projects Agency

DCCB	Digital Current Controlling Block
DC-EXCCII	Digitally Controllable Extra-X Second Generation Current Conveyor
DCW	Digital Control Word
DCWC	Digital Control Word Circuitry
DGTFET	Double Gate Tunnel Field Effect Transistor
DIBL	Drain Induced Barrier Lowering
DMDGDM	Duel Material Double Gate Dielectric Modulated
DMGAATFET	Dual Material Gate All Around Tunnel Field Effect Transistor
DNN	Deep Neural Network
DPCCII	Digitally Programmable Second Generation Current Conveyor
DPCFA	Digitally Programmable Current Feedback Amplifier
DPDVCC	Digitally Programmable Differential Voltage Current Conveyor
DUT	Device Under Test
DV-EXCCCII	Differential Volatge Extra-X Current Controlled Current Conveyor
ECG	Electro Cardio Graph
ECG	Electrocardiogram
EDA	Electronic Design Automation
EFBG	Etched Fiber Bragg Grating
EXCCII	Extra-X Second Generation Current Conveyor
FAD	Flavin Adenine Dinucleotide
FBG	Fiber Bragg Grating
FEDMGAA	Ferro Electric Dual Material Gate All Around
FET	Field-Effect Transistor
FSCV	Fast-Scan Cyclic Voltammetry
FWHM	Full Width Half Maximum
GAA	Gate All Around
GBR	Gradient Boosting
GCAPF	Gain Controllable All Pass Filter
GC-DMGJL	Graded Channel Dual Material Gate Junction Less
GIDL	Gate Induced Drain Lowering
GNN	Graph Neural Network
GNPs	Gold-Nanoparticles
GPR	Gaussian Process Regression
GPU	Graphics Processing Unit
GRAIDS	Gastrointestinal Artificial Intelligence Diagnostic System
HBM	High Bandwidth Memory
HE	Hemagglutinin Esterase
HEMT	High Electron Mobility Transistor
HfO_2	Hafnium Oxide

HP	High Pass
HRTEM	High Resolution Transmission Electron Microscopy
HSPICE	H(Hewlett)-Simulation Program with Integrated Circuit Emphasis
IC	Integrated Circuit
IDE	Inter-Digitated Electrodes
IL	Interleukin
ISF	Interstitial Fluid
IUPAC	International Union of Pure and Applied Chemistry
JL DG MOSFET	Junction Less Double Gate Metal Oxide Semiconductor Field Effect Transistor
JLDGTFET	junction Less Double Gate Tunnel Field Effect Transistor
KGD	Known Good Die
KNN	K-Nearest Neighbour
LP	Low Pass
LPG	Long Period Grating
LR	Linear Regression
MARS	Multivariate Adaptive Regression Splines
MATLAB	Matrix Laboratory
MgZnO	Magnesium Zinc Oxide
ML	Machine Learning
MLP	Multilayer Perceptron
MNP	Magnetic Nanoparticles
MOF	Metal-Organic Framework
MOSFET	Metal Oxide Field Effect Transistor
MOSFET	Metal Oxide Semiconductor Field Effect Transistor
MR	Multiple Regression
MWCNTs	Multi-Walled Carbon Nanotubes
NAD	Nicotinamide Adenine Dinucleotide
NCR	National Capital Region
NiNPs	Nickel Hexa-Cyanoferrate Nanoparticles
NMOS	N- channel Metal Oxide Semiconductor
NP	Nanoparticles
OPC	Optical Proximity Correction
PB	Phosphate Buffer
PCA	Principal Component Analysis
PCB	Printed Circuit Board
PDMS	Polydimethylsiloxane
PET	Polyethylene Terephthalate
PMOS	P-Channel Metal Oxide Semiconductor
POFBG	Polymer Optical Fiber Bragg Grating
PPA	Power, Performance and Area
PSPICE	Personal Simulation Program with Integrated Circuit Emphasis
QD	Quantum Dot

RBF	Radial Basis Function
RF	Radio Frequency
rGO	reduced Graphene Oxide
RISC V	Reduced Instruction Set Compute
RL	Reinforcement Learning
RNA	Ribonucleic Acid
RNN	Recurrent Neural Network
SARS	Severe Acute Respiratory Syndrome
SARS-CoV-2	Severe Acute Respiratory Syndrome Coronavirus 2
SCE	Short Channel Effect
SEM	Scanning Electron Microscope
SiO_2	Silicon Dioxide
SOC	System On Chip
SOI	Silicon On Insulator
SPR	Surface Plasmon Resonance
SRH	Shockley-Read-Hall
SVM	Support Vector Machine
SVR	Support Vector Regression
SWCNTs	Single-Walled Carbon Nanotubes
TCAD	Technology Computer Aided Design
TFET	Tunnel Field Effect Transistor
TIR	Total Internal Reflection
TMD	Transition Metal Dichalcogenide
TMM	Transfer Matrix Method
TOC	Total Organic Carbon
UF	Universal Filter
UG-DMGJL	Uniform Channel Dual Material Gate Junction Less
UTI	Urinary Tract Infection
UV	Ultra Voilet
VGG	Visual Geometry Group
VLSI	Very Large-Scale Integration
VM	Voltage Mode
VT	Threshold Voltage
WEKA	Waikato Environment for Knowledge Analysis
WHO	World Health Organization
ZnO	Zinc Oxide
ZnSe	Zinc Selenide

Chapter 1

Enhancement of Dynamic Range of Surface Plasmon Resonance (SPR) Biosensor Using High Refractive Index Prism

A Theoretical Approach

Akash Srivastava
KNIPSS Sultanpur, Uttar Pradesh, India

Sajal Agarwal
Rajiv Gandhi Institute of Petroleum Technology, Jais, India

CONTENTS

ABBREVIATIONS

BRE   Bio recognition element
FWHM   Full width half maximum
IUPAC   International Union of Pure and Applied Chemistry
SPR   Surface plasmon resonance
TIR   Total internal reflection
TMD   Transition metal dichalcogenide
TMM   Transfer Matrix Method
ZnSe   Zinc selenide

DOI: 10.1201/9781003431138-1

1

1.1 INTRODUCTION

Optical sensing [1], optoelectronics [2], and photonic devices [3] are the most significant emerging fields from the last four decades, and they continue to grow in terms of invention, innovation and research [4]. The essential requirement for a biosensor is that bacterial detection should be exclusive, sensitive and provide a rapid response. Those sensors which are actively operating in business are very steeply-priced, and furthermore they need consumable sensor chips, which have to encompass a few essential specifications aiming for much smaller size, much smaller thickness, a powerful sensing vicinity and so on. Biosensors determine the presence and concentration of specific biological substances in biological analytes, and their key components are bioreceptors and transducers. Bioreceptors or ligands may be enzymes, proteins or antibodies; while transducers convert biochemical activity into electrical energy. Similarly they are sensing elements for gas-sensing of hazardous gases like methane, carbon dioxide, or rogen among others [5]. Professor Leland C Clark Jnr (1918–2005) is known as the "father of biosensors", and the present-day glucose sensor, used daily by millions of diabetic patients, is based on his research idea [6]. Sensors that support the surface plasmon resonance (SPR) development were projected initially in 1983 by Liedberg et al. [7] to measure the refractive index of organic layers adsorbate on a thin metal film. Since that time, SPR has been widely used as a detection technique in chemical and biochemical sensing, pharmaceutical analysis and environmental monitoring. In an SPR sensor, a change in the refractive index of a test sample (called an analyte) changes the coupling conditions between incident light and surface plasmon waves propagating along the metal-analyte interface. This change can be measured as a change in one of the characteristics of the output light wave. Surface plasmon resonance sensors are excellent for gas and liquid analysis as well as for measuring temperature, humidity, chemical and biological composition. This is because these parameters change the refractive index of the analyte. As defined by the International Union of Pure and Applied Chemistry (IUPAC), "a biosensor is a stand-alone, integrated device that can provide specific quantitative or semi-quantitative analytical tools using biological recognition elements (biochemical receptors) that are in direct spatial contact with the transducer element" [8]. Surface plasmon resonance sensors have gained enormous interest for their biosensing applications, for example the finding of DNA, proteins, antibody-antigen connections, cells and bacteria. Their unparalleled excellence in real-time monitoring and high sensitivity, as well as having no necessity for fluorescent labeling and being resistant in contradiction of electromagnetic interferences make them superior. In the last two decades, plasmonics have played a major role in nanophotonics and particularly in sensing, due to providing extreme sensitivity and reliability. Plasmon is a combined oscillation of those electrons which are supplied on the metallic surface, and are excited when treated with an electromagnetic wave. Surface plasmon is propagating in nature; when a monochromatic light is incident at the metal-dielectric interface, their energy carried through the photons is transferred to the SPs, and this phenomenon is referred to as surface plasmon resonance (SPR). Drude proposed a microscopic explanation of the dynamics of electrons in metals in classical terms, and obtained the equation of motion of a damped oscillator, in which electrons move between heavier and relatively fixed background ions. The Drude-Sommerfeld model [9] of the free electron gas is determined by Equation 1.1:

$$m_e \frac{\partial^2 r}{\partial t^2} + m_e \gamma_d \frac{\partial r}{\partial t} = eE_0 e^{-i\omega t} \tag{1.1}$$

Where γ_d relates to a damping term, m_e (mass of effective free electrons) is a charge on free electrons and E_0 and ω are amplitude and frequency of incident light. A prism is required to increase the wave vector of the incident light to match the wave vector of the surface plasmon. In the category of various types of prism (like SF10, SF11, SF5, BAK1, BK7, 2S2G, BAF10, etc.), a BK7 prism is frequently used, due to its low refractive index (n = 1.51) and it has been confirmed as an exceptional substrate with high sensitivity. BK7 features brilliant transmission at wavelengths from 350 nm to 2000 nm, good thermal extension, low price, tough glass and good chemical resistance. A borosilicate, silica and acrylate glass based rectangular prism (most commonly BK7) is used in the visible region because of its sensing-friendly properties like excellent transmission, low refractive index (1.51), less scattering behavior and robustness [10].

1.2 SOLUTION OF SURFACE PLASMON WAVE FOR MULTIPLE LAYERS USING TRANSFER MATRIX METHOD (TMM)

If the sensor structure contains a single layer or two layers, its reflectance and transmittance values can be estimated using Fresnel's equation [11], which proves to be a difficult technique for multi-layer, thin-film structures. The transfer matrix method (TMM) [12] is a suitable method for estimating reflectance and transmittance values for sensing models containing N-layer.

The tangential field between the boundaries is related by Equation 1.2:

$$\left[A_1 \, B_1 \right] = M_2 \, M_3 M_4 \ldots \ldots M_{N-1} \left[A_{N-1} \, B_{N-1} \right] = M \left[A_{N-1} \, B_{N-1} \right] \tag{1.2}$$

Here, A_1 and B_1 are the tangential components of electric and magnetic field separately at the boundary of the first layer likewise A_{N-1} and B_{N-1} are the tangential components of electric and magnetic fields correspondingly at the edge of the Nth layer. M is the characteristic matrix of the collective structure, given by

$$M = \prod_{K=2}^{N-1} M_K = \left[M_{11} \, M_{12} \, M_{21} \, M_{22} \right] \tag{1.3}$$

Here,

$$M_K = \left[\cos \beta_k - \sin \left(\frac{\beta_k}{q_k} \right) - i q_k \sin \beta_k \cos \beta_k \right], \tag{1.4}$$

$$q_k = \left(\frac{\mu_k}{\varepsilon_k} \right)^{\frac{1}{2}} \cos \theta_k$$

and

$$\beta_k = \frac{2\pi}{\lambda} n_k \cos \theta_k \left(d_k \right)$$

The amplitude reflection coefficient (r) and reflectivity (R) for p-polarized light obtained by following some mathematical steps as

$$R = |r|^2 = \frac{\left(M_{11} + M_{12} q_N \right) q_1 - \left(M_{21} + M_{22} q_N \right)}{\left(M_{11} + M_{12} q_N \right) q_1 + \left(M_{21} + M_{22} q_N \right)} \tag{1.5}$$

1.2.1 Prism Coupling

Otto (1968) and Kretschmann (1971) developed an optical prism coupling scheme for SPR excitation using the "total internal reflection (TIR)" concept. Prism-based SPR biosensors are mainly based on two well-known configurations: the Otto configuration and the Kretschmann configuration (see Figure 1.1). In the Otto method, there is an air gap between the metal and the TIR surface (Figure 1.1a). However, while detecting SPR in a solid-state environment may be an appropriate method, maintaining the distance between the metal and the TIR surface is a tedious task and at the same time reduces the effectiveness of the SPR, making it less useful.

In the Kretschmann configuration, the metal layer is in direct contact with the prism, making it an economical method of plasmon generation. Figure 1.1b represents the Kretschmann configuration.

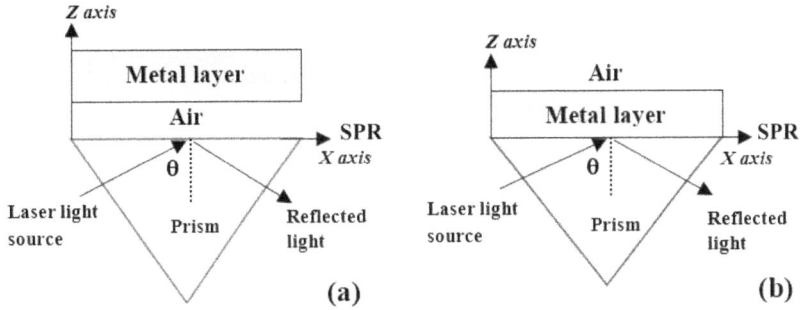

Figure 1.1 Schematic of realizing the SPR plasmon resonance idea. (a) Otto configuration. (b) Kretschmann configuration.

1.2.2 Effect of Prism Refractive Index on Resonance Angle Position

The selection of prism is very important for efficient sensing because it directly affects the position of SPR angle dip. As we know the SPR equation is written as:

$$n_p \sin \theta_{sp} = \mathrm{Re}\left(\sqrt{\frac{\varepsilon_m \varepsilon_d}{\varepsilon_m + \varepsilon_d}} \right) \tag{1.6}$$

Where n_p is prism refractive index, ε_d or n_d^2 is refractive index of dielectric medium, ε_m is the dielectric constant of metal and θ_{sp} is the SPR angle. 'Re' denotes the real part of the term in parentheses. In order to satisfy Equation 1.1,the following condition must be satisfied to get $\sin\theta_{sp} < 1$

$$\left(\sqrt{\frac{\varepsilon_m \varepsilon_d}{\varepsilon_m + \varepsilon_d}} \right) < 90° \tag{1.7}$$

Due to this condition, it's necessary to select the prism which has a high refractive index in comparison to the refractive index of dielectric medium [11]. The higher the value of n_p, the lower will be the θ_{sp}. Now, let n_d is ~1.45 or more, then, according to above condition n_p, the value should be more than 1.6. Thus, in practice, for a glass prism with n_p a value in the range 1.7–1.8 is selected. Working with a high n_p value, the θ_{sp} value lies in the low angle region of 40–50°.

1.3 DYNAMIC RANGE ENHANCEMENT THEORETICAL ANALYSIS

Despite all these properties, there is a major issue of a very short dynamic range for sensing the water-based biosamples. If limit of detection is minimum concentration/amount of the analyte which can be sensed then the range between limit of detection and minimum concentration which can be measured with confidence is nothing but the dynamic range of sensor. For a conventional SPR sensor, involving Au as a metal layer, the resonance angle θ_{spr} lies at ~74° which is already very high. As with water, the working refractive index span possible is from 1.33 to 1.47, so for high refractive index variation SPR shift monitoring is very limited for a small range. This situation constrains the user to limited sensing application. To overcome the issue, for a mean high refractive index based dielectric sample and, for a large dynamic range a very common approach is to apply a prism of the higher refractive index because practically it excites surface plasmon as well as reducing θ_{spr}. This will facilitate the user's greater angular span and allow more solvent hosts to be used. A high refractive index (RI) prism made up from calcium fluoride (CaF2), or zinc selenide (ZnSe) is a replacement for the most commonly used borosilicate-based prism. It has been observed that an SPR sensor using a high RI prism exhibits very much less shift in SPR angle, and hence, has low sensitivity. Still, the advantage is that the obtained SPR angle is sharp, and one can observe a large value of difference of refractive index from its reference value. For example, by using a ZnSe prism-based SPR sensor a user can observe the change in refractive index from the span of 1.33 to 1.7 [13]. From an analysis point of view, we have taken a very simple Kretschmann configuration based SPR sensor model where, in the flow cell, the sample under consideration is filled. A graphical analysis is given for the proposed conventional model of SPR sensor by using MATLAB software comparing the low refractive index borosilicate prism to the high RI-based ZnSe prism in Figure 1.2(a) and (b), and also shows the proposed sensing device is capable of biosample for a large RI span. For analysis purposes, the authors have taken pure water, with

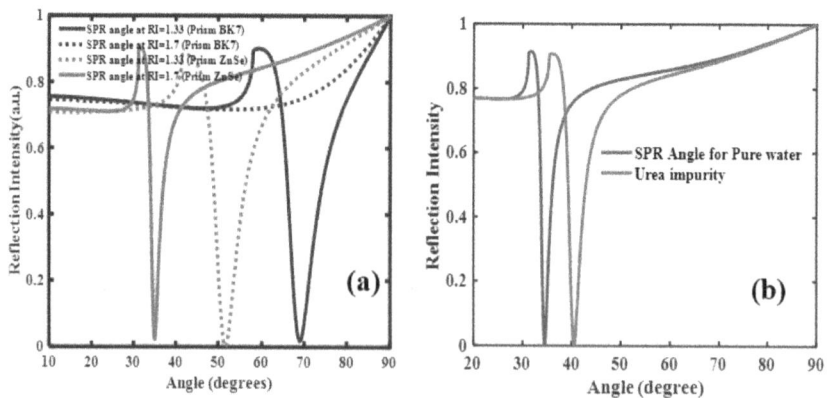

Figure 1.2 (a) Comparison study of the dynamic range of a conventional SPR sensor from 1.33 to 1.7 refractive index span, for sensing purpose: the blue curve is for a BK7 borosilicate glass prism-based sensor, and brown SPR curve is for a ZnSe prism-based SPR sensor. (b) The large span of refractive index variation (1.33–1.48) for urea detection.

a refractive index of 1.33, and a urea mixed liquid sample having a refractive index of 1.48. It can be observed that the proposed sensor is able to detect the urea-based impurity by means of a shifting in SPR angle; the sensitivity of the conventional sensor is calculated as 36.8°/RIU which is not remarkable and can be increased by applying some 2D materials [14], or a heterostructure of 2D/ TMD materials on top of the metal layer [15].

1.4 COMPARATIVE PERFORMANCE ANALYSIS OF SPR SENSORS BY TAKING DIFFERENT HIGH REFRACTIVE PRISMS

From Table 1.1 it can be observed that to enhance the dynamic range for those samples which have a high refractive index from their reference value, the prism having a high refractive index is useful. We have given two analyses of sensitivity: in the first column for conventional structure, and in another column, we observe that sensitivity increases when a metal layer is functionalized with a 2D/TMD heterostructure (in a stack with each other). The reason is that as a bio recognition element (BRE) we applied a graphene monolayer, which provided favorable conditions for biosensing, like a high surface-to-volume ratio, a honeycomb lattice structure in a monolayer surface, high electron mobility and, most important, stability in an ambient environment. Also, MoS_2 has a thickness-dependent tunable bandgap (metal to semiconductor property) and a high absorption property of photons [16]. A thin layer of silicon (Si) over the metal surface is used to improve the sensitivity of the SPR sensor, since it increases the field intensity of the excitation light at the silicon-sensing layer interface [17]. The field intensity at dielectric interfaces increases, due to which the excitation of SPs is enhanced because of the high absorption behavior of the metal and silicon layer. The study is given in Table 1.2 and in inset the modified structure is given. Detailed graphical study is given in Figure 1.3 where the sensitivity analysis when using different prisms is given.

Table 1.1 Sensitivity analysis for conventional structure and including 2D/TMD heterostructure

	Types of prism	Refractive index	Sensitivity for conventional structure (1.33–1.7)	Sensitivity with 2D/TMD heterostructure (1.33–1.7)
1.	2s2g prism	2.358	48.45	52.02
2.	ZnSe	2.57	41.02	43.67
3.	Boron Phosphide	3.00	31.91	33.75
4.	Gallium Phosphide (GaP)	3.3	27.86	29.24
5.	Cadmium germanium phosphide (CdGeP$_2$)	3.48	25.83	27.40

Table 1.2 Enhancement of sensitivity by including silicon as an interlayer between sensing medium and metal layer

Types of prism	Sensitivity with 2D/TMD heterostructure and silicon as interlayer (1.33–1.7)
1. 2s2g prism	81.13
2. ZnSe	72.45
3. Boron Phosphide	50.78
4. GaP [18]	42.89
5. Cadmium germanium phosphide (CdGeP₂)	40.27

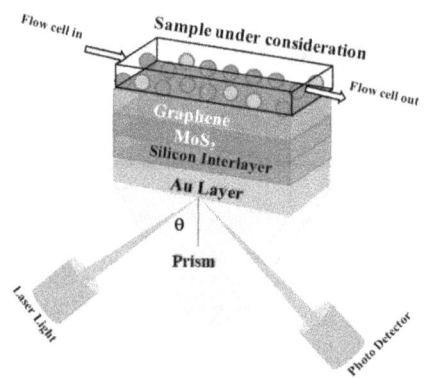

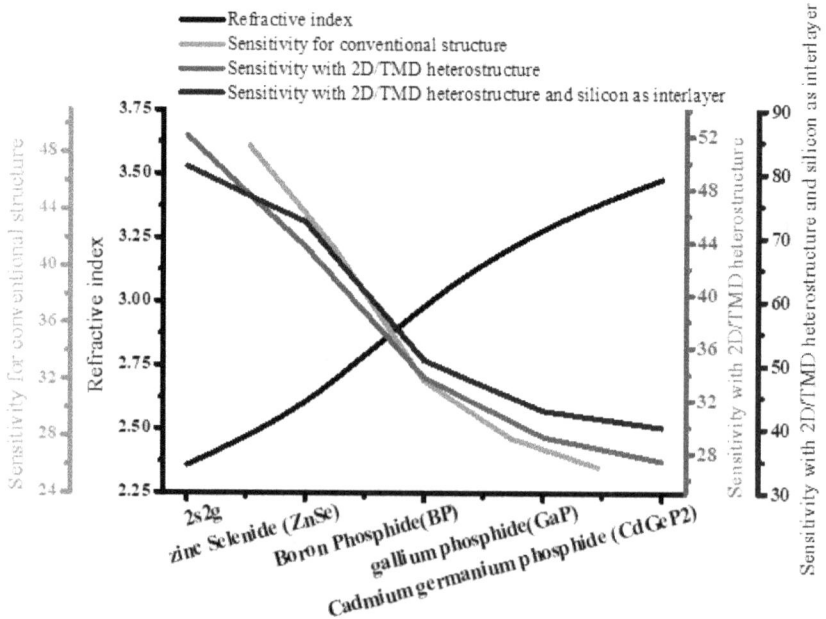

Figure 1.3 Comparative performance analysis of various SPR based sensor using different high refractive prisms to enhance dynamic range.

The dynamic range of an SPR sensor with a low refractive index prism can be increased as suggested by Probowo et al. [19]. They show in their paper that if aluminum (Al) is used as a metallic layer it is possible to increase the dynamic range up to 1.45 refractive index of sample. An Al-based sensor provides high penetration depth compared to silver and gold. However, Al is not a good option to replace gold, first, because it oxidizes earlier in the ambient environment and second, for those samples that are acidic in nature with a high pH value, Al is reactive so it can affect the originality of sample. As a solution to this issue, a gold coating is applied directly on Al.

1.5 CONCLUSION

In this chapter the authors have given an overview of surface plasmon resonance-based techniques and their application in various kinds of sensing applications. The major components of a biosensor and how SPR technique plays a significant role in biosensing applications are shown here. Dynamic range is a very important parameter in sensors, and the possible ways to increase the dynamic range and how a prism's refractive index is useful in dynamic range modulation have been demonstrated in this chapter.

REFERENCES

1. S. Kumar and R. Singh, "Recent optical sensing technologies for the detection of various biomolecules: Review," *Optics & Laser Technology*, vol. 134, p. 106620, Feb. 2021.
2. A. Rogers and V. Handerek, "An introduction to optoelectronics," *Handbook of Optoelectronics* CRC Press, pp. 3–20, Oct. 2017.
3. I. Amiri, S. Azzuhri, M. Jalil, H. Hairi, J. Ali, M. Bunruangses, and P. Yupapin, "Introduction to photonics: Principles and the most recent applications of microstructures," *Micromachines*, vol. 9, no. 9, p. 452, Sep. 2018.
4. D. E. Bloom and D. Cadarette, "Infectious disease threats in the twenty-first century: strengthening the global response," *Frontiers in Immunology*, vol. 10, p. 549, Mar. 2019.
5. R. C. Chatelier, T. R. Gengenbach, H. J. Griesser, M. Brighamburke, and D. J. Oshannessy, "A general method to recondition and reuse Biacore sensor chips fouled with covalently immobilized protein/peptide," *Analytical Biochemistry*, vol. 229, no. 1, pp. 112–118, Jul. 1995.
6. J. Homola, "Present and future of surface Plasmon resonance biosensors," *Analytical and Bioanalytical Chemistry*, vol. 377, no. 3, pp. 528–539, 2003.
7. B. Liedberg, C. Nylander, and I. Lunström, "Surface plasmon resonance for gas detection and biosensing," *Sensors and Actuators*, vol. 4, pp. 299–304, Jan. 1983.
8. B. Jurado-Sánchez, "Nanoscale biosensors based on self-propelled objects," *Biosensors*, vol. 8, no. 3, p. 59, Jun. 2018.

9. Z. He, F. Li, Y. Liu, F. Yao, L. Xu, X. Han, and K. Wang, "Principle and applications of the coupling of surface plasmons and excitons," *Applied Sciences*, vol. 10, no. 5, p. 1774, Mar. 2020.

10. D. Pines and J. R. Schrieffer, "Approach to equilibrium of electrons, plasmons, and phonons in quantum and classical plasmas," *Physical Review*, vol. 125, no. 3, pp. 804–812, Feb. 1962.

11. G. Gupta, M. Sugimoto, Y. Matsui, and J. Kondoh, "Use of a low refractive index prism in surface plasmon resonance biosensing," *Sensors and Actuators B: Chemical*, vol. 130, no. 2, pp. 689–695, Mar. 2008.

12. Widayanti, K. A. K. and A. B. Utomo, "A comparative study of applying different prisms an metalic layers in the surface plasmon resonance-based biosensor enhanced by the inclusion of the core-shell nanoparticles," *International Conference on Science and Applied Science (ICSAS) 2018*, 2018.

13. J. Canning, J. Qian et.al. "Large dynamic range SPR measurements using a ZnSe prism," *Photonic Sensors*, vol. 5, no. 3, pp. 278–283, 2015.

14. Akash Srivastava and Y. K. Prajapati "Performance analysis of silicon and BluePhosphorene/MoS2 hetero- structure based SPR sensor," *Photonic Sensors*, vol. 9, no. 33, pp 1–9, Feb. 2019.

15. Akash Srivastava, Alka Verma, Ritwick Das, and Y. K. Prajapati, "A theoretical approach to improve the performance of SPR biosensor using MXene and black phosphorus," *Optik - International Journal for Light and Electron Optics*, vol.203, pp. 1–9, 2020.

16. A. Srivastava, A. Verma, and Y. K. Prajapati, "Effect of 2D, TMD, perovskite, and 2D transition metal carbide/nitride materials on performance parameters of SPR biosensor," *Handbook of Nanomaterials for Sensing Applications*, Elsevier, pp. 57–90, 2021.

17. M. Bruna and S. Borini, "Optical constants of graphene layers in the visible range," *Applied Physics Letter*, vol. 94, no. 3, pp. 4–13, 2009.

18. A. K. Mishra, S. K. Mishra, and R. K. Verma, "An SPR-based sensor with an extremely large dynamic range of refractive index measurements in the visible region," *Journal of Physics D: Applied Physics*, vol. 48, no. 43, p. 435502, Oct. 2015.

19. B. A. Prabowo, I. D. P. Hermida, R. V. Manurung, A. Purwidyantri, and K.-C. Liu, "Nano-film aluminum-gold for ultra-high dynamic-range surface plasmon resonance chemical sensor," *Frontiers of Optoelectronics*, vol. 12, no. 3, pp. 286–295, Apr. 2019.

Chapter 2

Introduction to Fiber Bragg Grating Sensors for Liquid Sensing Applications

Fiber Bragg Grating Sensors for Liquid Sensing

Shivangi Srivastava and Sajal Agarwal

Rajiv Gandhi Institute of Petroleum Technology, Jais, India

CONTENTS

ABBREVIATIONS

EFBG	Etched fiber Bragg grating
FBG	Fiber Bragg grating
FWHM	Full width half maximum
LPG	Long period grating
POFBG	Polymer optical fiber Bragg grating
UV	Ultraviolet

2.1 INTRODUCTION

In the last decade many mechanical, electrical, and optical sensors have been used for level detection [1–5]. Fiber Bragg grating (FBG) based sensors have become prominent since they have various advantages over other sensors. Optical sensors are inherently dielectric and non-conductive when compared with traditional sensors. An FBG is used for liquid sensing, hence it is applicable to fuel storage and biochemical systems. This is possible due to its passivity and multiplexing. In 1978, Ken Hill demonstrated the fiber Bragg grating, which is basically created by doing periodic and aperiodic

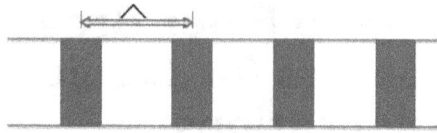

Figure 2.1 Construction of FBG.

perturbation of the refractive index in the core of the optical fiber in the direction of propagation. The refractive index perturbation leads to a reflection of light (specific wavelength). So, this full system can be treated as an optical filter, where it blocks a specific wavelength of light.

Figure 2.1 shows the variation of the refractive index in the direction of propagation. Here the darker part has a higher refractive index than the lighter one. Hence, it can be used as a sensing application by blocking certain wavelengths.

The variation of refractive index in the core of the optical fiber is known as the FBG and thus, optical fiber makes a stable sensor. Now, if any strain is applied over this variation, it further changes in the proportion to strain. It creates a shift in wavelength due to reflection. Thus, measurement was performed by using the fiber Bragg grating. When light propagates through the fiber Bragg grating, a specific light beam is reflected by the refractive index. This reflective wavelength is known as "Bragg wavelength".

Although Hill discovered the concept of FBG and that the grating spectrum is the function of temperature and strain, at that time the fiber was very lossy. This limited FBG for practical application. In 1989, three scientists, Meltz, Morey and Glenn [7], made great improvements (such as side writing of FBGs outside of fibers and FBGs as mirrors for fiber laser cavities, and also as pigtailed output couplers for semiconductor lasers) [8–10]. In 1993, phase mask and hydrogen loading were discovered which made FBGs more useful for practical implementation. In the 20th century, the periodic modification in the reflective index of the fiber's core was defined as microstructure. If light hits this periodic microstructure within the fiber, a specific wavelength of light is reflected but other than that all wavelengths will pass.

When coming to sensing, a polymer fiber Bragg grating is better than the normal silica fiber since it has excellent flexibility, higher mechanical resistance, low cost, ruggedness and many more although it is having higher transmission loss.

Basically, fiber Bragg grating is written by placing the fiber in ultraviolet light radiation. An interference pattern produced when the UV light falls over the fiber. Due to this, there will be permanent damage (change) in the refractive index (see Figure 2.2). Hence, a periodic perturbation in the refractive index of the fiber's core is obtained. The number of wavelengths reflected is dependent on the refractive index variation. All reflected signals affect constructively and add up to a wavelength known as the "Bragg wavelength".

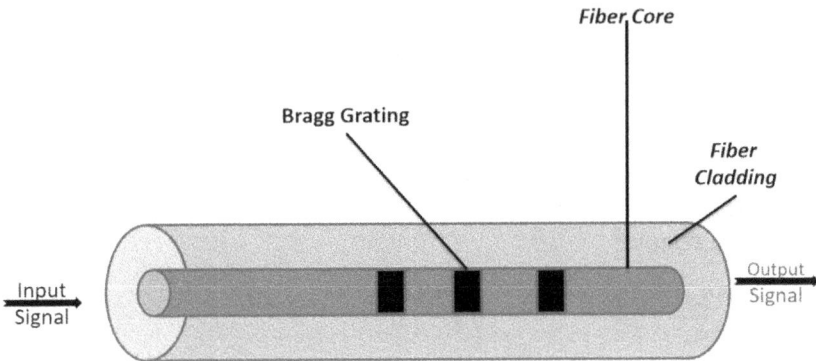

Figure 2.2 Working of a fiber Bragg grating.

2.2 PRINCIPLES OF FIBER BRAGG GRADING

A periodic or aperiodic change in the structure of a material is known as a grating. This concept is used in optical fiber, where the refractive index of the core varies, and this variation causes the reflection of a specific wavelength of light. The number of wavelengths is depended on the amount of variation in the refractive index. Bragg grating was discovered by William Bragg. The basic physics behind Bragg grating is when a light beam travels between two layers of objects (or two layers of materials), there is a phase difference between them. Such phase difference produces constructive interference and, thus, the reflection of specific wavelengths is obtained.

In short, when a light wave propagates along the fiber Bragg grating, there will be reflection of specific wavelengths and transmission of all other wavelengths. The wavelength of the combined signal of all the reflected waves is known as the Bragg wavelength. An incident light wave is reflected if it satisfies the condition:

$$\lambda_{Bragg} = 2n_{eff}\Lambda \qquad\qquad (2.1)$$

where
   λ_{Bragg}: the wavelength of reflected light wave (Bragg wavelength)
   n_{eff}: index of refraction (average of core and grating area's refractive index)
   Λ: period of grating

Equation 2.1 is known as the Bragg relation. The FBG sensors measure different quantities (such as pressure, strain and temperature) by calculating the shift in Bragg wavelength since Equation 2.1 shows that Bragg wavelength is dependent on the period of grating and net refractive index. So, by applying the measuring quantity onto the fiber Bragg grating, these two parameters were affected, and thus, the Bragg wavelength shifted. For proper working of the grating the following conditions or phenomena must be satisfied:

- The wavelength of the incident and reflected light beam must be the same ($\lambda_{wf} = \lambda_{wi}$).
- The direction of the diffracted wave vector is opposite to the incident wave vector.

$$2 \frac{2\pi n_{eff}}{\lambda_{Bragg}} = \frac{2\pi}{\Lambda} \tag{2.2}$$

- The wave vector of the scattered radiation k_f is equal to the addition of the grating wave vector k and incident wave vector k_i ($k_i + k = k_f$).
- Reflection of some wavelength from the grading edge happens. The reason behind this is Fresnel's reflection.
- This can be described in other words as when a light beam travels from one certain refractive index to a different refractive index. Both reflection and refraction occur.
- When perfectly polarized light is transmitted with a particular incident angle through a transparent dielectric surface (e.g., core-cladding interface), there will be no reflection.

When an unpolarized wave at the same angle is incident, it is reflected from the surface, and this angle is known as Brewster's angle.

- When the light is incident onto the crystal surface, its angle of incident Θ, will reflect back with the same angle of scattering. Constructive interference will occur when the path difference d is equal to the total number of wavelength incident, and Bragg condition satisfaction is given by Equation 2.3:

$$n\lambda = 2d \sin\Theta \tag{2.3}$$

where
   n: number of wavelength
   d: distance between two planes
   λ : wavelength of incident wave
   Θ: angle of incident

2.3 LIQUID SENSING VIA DIFFERENT STRUCTURES

As discussed earlier, the FBG is used for different sensing applications. Much research is done in the field of these sensors since they have a server advantage over the other sensors. Liquid-level sensing is crucial for many applications such as: measuring the concentration of different chemicals in the fuel and biochemical industry, or monitoring and regulating the flow of different liquids in various industries and different plants. Before the development of optical sensors, electro-mechanical sensors were used for liquid sensing. But, due to safety concerns, optical sensors are the better option. Optical fiber sensors have high accuracy, are compact in size, cost-effective, and multiplexing of signals is easy in comparison with traditional sensors [11]. The first liquid-level fiber sensor, where grating is done at the tip of sensor, was developed by Spenner. With the development of the Fabry-Perot interferometer proposed by Wang, a large range continuous sensor was developed [12]. In this device, a fabrication process is used by CO_2 laser-heating, fusion-bonding technology. There are different types of liquid sensor configuration, such as: a polished angular fiber end face, fiber bending and incorporation of a prism and fibers [13], cladding removed fiber devices [14–19], fiber Bragg grating (FBG) [20–26] and long period grating (LPG)-based platforms [27–33]. When the sensor's tip comes out from the measured liquid, the refractive index surrounding the tip changes, hence reflected light intensity changes. Various fiber liquid sensors have been investigated in recent years with different working principles [11, 34–36]. The refractive index or the grating period can be varied in the structure of the FBG. Although grating is the periodic variation in the refractive index, but it is not always true. It can be varied according to variations in physical parameters. So, according to the structure, the following types of grating are available, which can also be used for liquid sensing.

1. **Uniform Grating**: In uniform Bragg grating, there will be periodically changing layers of refractive index. Uniform Bragg is defined by a uniform period and constant period of change in the refractive index. It is also known as "reflection grating". For this type of grating refractive index, the profile is given by Equation 2.4:

$$n(z) = n_{core} + \Delta n_o A(z) n_d(z) \tag{2.4}$$

where
$n_d(z)$: index variation function
$A(z)$: apodization function (For uniform grating: $A(z) = 1$)
n_{core}: core refractive index
Δn_o: maximum index variation

If we apply strain or temperature externally on the grating, then we are able to make different types of grating. When light travels through the grating, it reflects back from the dark section as shown in Figure 2.3. The black part has a greater refractive index than the white part.

Figure 2.3 Uniform grating.

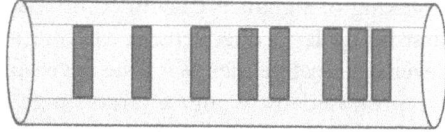

Figure 2.4 Chirped grating.

In the output characteristics, the side lobe and relative power are increased, if the length of grating increases. But the side lobes are not desirable. So, we need to trade off. These parameters are also affected by increasing modulation depth. An increment in modulation depth also increases full width-half maximum (FWHM).

2. **Chirped Fiber Grating:** In chirped FBGs, variation of refractive index is not uniform. It can be linear or non-linear. The grating period changes linearly along the axis of fiber in linear chirp, whereas in non-linear chirp it varies non-linearly. Due to the non-uniform grating, each component of wavelength is reflected at different positions, hence, it adds dispersion. It leads to different delay times for different reflected wavelengths. It introduces different group delays which are dependent on wavelength. So, it enables the dispersion compensation [37–41]. In a chirped grating (see Figure 2.4), a physical quantity like temperature or pressure is applied over the section of the grating, unlike in a uniform grating where temperature or pressure is applied over the whole grating length [42]. So, it can be used for detecting hotspots [43], and strain discontinuities [44].

3. **Long Period Grating:** In this type of structure, light couples from guided mode into forward propagating cladding mode. But, due to a lot of absorption and scattering, the wave is lost. Basically, in LPG the refractive index changes in some periodic manner (from 100 micrometers to millimeter) [11]. Due to this, core mode is coupled with a number of cladding modes. At the resonance wavelength, if the coupling coefficient and pitch along the grating are changed, a phase shift is obtained along the grating. This resonance wavelength is when the coupling is strongest between the specific radiation mode (cladding mode) and guided mode. Optical fiber LPG structure consists of a three-layer cylindrical waveguide structure with core, cladding and

ambient surroundings [12–14]. This is widely used for chemical sensing.

4. **Sampled Grating**: Although it is difficult to vary Bragg wavelength across the fiber, it can be easily controlled by adjusting the period of sampled grating. This is uniform periodic grating at different sampled regions.

5. **Tilted Fiber Grating**: In tilted FBG, modification of refractive index is tilted at a particular angle to the core of fiber axis, unlike standard FBG. Reflected wavelength and bandwidth depend on a tilted angle. It is used for multimode sensors.

6. **Apodized Fiber Bragg Grating**: In uniform grating, variation of refractive index is uniform. But side lobes are the problem present at the adjacent wavelength. Side lobes are not desirable in the output. So, we need to minimize the side lobes by using different mathematical gratings such as cosine, raised cosine, tanh, blackman, gassiuan and so forth. This is known as apodization grating. Some examples of the mathematical gratings are:

- **Cosine Grating**: Here modulation of the grating is based on the cosine function. It is an example of non-uniform grating which is suitable for liquid-sensing applications. It gives better results than uniform grating. The refractive index modulation function is given by Equation 2.5:

$$n(z) = n_{core} + \Delta n_0 n_d(z) A(z) \tag{2.5}$$

where

$$A(Z) = \cos\frac{\pi z}{2a} \tag{2.6}$$

It is clear from the mathematical relation that grating is modulated according to the cosine function. It is better than uniform grating. Here, in cosine grating, although side lobes are there, they have less relative power.

- **Raised Cosine Grating**: This type of grating function is a compromise between hanning and hamming window. To reduce side lobes, a raised cosine grating is used, and thus, the bandwidth reduces. The refractive index modulation function is given by Equation 2.7:

$$n(z) = n_{core} + \Delta n_0 n_d(z) A(z) \tag{2.7}$$

where

$$A(z) = \cos^n \Theta \tag{2.8}$$

If we compare the raised cosine and cosine gratings, the raised cosine grating has less reflective power, and more FWHM but fewer (almost negligible for low value) side lobes. Raised cosine grating is useful for the long optical link since it has less crosstalk and inter-symbol interference.

- **Tanh Grating:** If the variation of the refractive index is according to the tan hyperbolic function of trigonometric, the grating is known as tanh grating. It has a different phase shift and greater bandwidth than the cosine and raised cosine gratings. The index varies from the beginning of the grating.Index variation function of grating is given by Equation 2.7:

$$n(z) = n_{core} + \Delta n_0 n_d(z) A(z) \tag{2.9}$$

where

$$A(z) = 1 + \tanh\left[T\left(1 - 2\left|\frac{\Theta}{\Pi}\right|^{\alpha}\right)\right] \tag{2.10}$$

Here, phase shift is different to the other trigonometric gratings. After the comparative analysis, the side lobes are less than for the cosine grating, but greater than for the raised cosine grating. So, it can be used for liquid sensing although the relative power is less than the cosine grating.

- **Blackman Grating:** For minimizing the side lobes, the Blackman window is a very effective function by which grating can be modulated. Here the apodization function for the Blackman window is given by Equation 2.11:

$$A(z) = \frac{1 + (1 + B)\cos(\Theta) + B\cos(2\Theta)}{2 + 2B} \tag{2.11}$$

where
B: controlling factor of the window

Now, the refractive index can be varied according to the apodization function, as shown in Equation 2.12, since:

$$n(z) = n_{core} + \Delta n_0 n_d(z) A(z) \tag{2.12}$$

In the Blackman grating, the side lobes are the same as in the cosine grating, relative power is the same as Tanh and the FWHM is less than the cosine grating.

The permanent and periodic change in the refractive index with the short period Λ along the direction of propagation is known as the FBG. This can be inscribed through ultraviolet light interference patterns, phase-mask inscription and point-to-point inscription (through femtosecond pulsed lasers). These are the silica fibers. To increase the throughput, inscription and favourable attenuation, another alternative is polymer fiber [47–49]. In polymer grating, basically, the material-based grating is done where the core is doped with different polymer for enhancement of photosensitivity, as introduced in 1999 [55]. Polymer optical Bragg grating has different material properties than silica, which has helped it gain popularity in various applications of sensing. Polymer has many advantages over silica fiber, such as more sensitivity toward temperature changes, a large range of wavelength tunability, and more flexibility among others. So, it can be useful for strain [52] and pressure sensors [53]. Basically, a polymer has sensitivity toward temperature that is double that of silica [54].

7. **Polymer Fiber Bragg Grating:** This is a great alternative to silica fiber. Polymer fiber Bragg grating is widely used for liquid sensing. It is done by applying strain on the silicone rubber diaphragm. Polymer FBG sensors have a linear response and good repeatability. The system consists of a diaphragm, which is dipped in the measuring liquid at one side, whereas the other side is fixed onto the cavity, which is filled with air whose pressure is same as the atmosphere [15]. Thus, the thickness of the diaphragm is deflected as the external pressure increases, which is dependent on the increment of the liquid level. This will create strain across the disk and this strain can be measured. The strain of the diaphragm (maximum at center) is linearly dependent on the change in liquid density. The deformation in the diaphragm will change the fiber dimension, which turns into Bragg wavelength λ_B. Due to deformation in disk, the shift in wavelength is given by Equation 2.13:

$$\Delta\lambda_B = \lambda_B \left(1 - \rho_e\right)\varepsilon_{\max} \tag{2.13}$$

where

ρ_e: photo-elastic coefficient of the fiber
$\varepsilon_{\max}$: maximum strain
λ_B: initial Bragg wavelength

Thus, change in liquid level can be monitored or measured by seeing the shift in Bragg wavelength. It can be further divided into single polymer optical fiber Bragg grating (POFBG) sensor and multi sensor-based system.

2.4 SOME PRACTICAL IMPLEMENTATIONS OF FIBER BRAGG GRATING AS SENSORS

Liquid sensing is a significant application of the fiber Bragg grating. Some of these practical implementations are given below:

Fuel Sensing: Adulteration in petroleum products is very common and results in pollution, and early damage to the engine and machine. Adulteration in petroleum products is done by mixing kerosene and other organic compounds, since they are cheaper than the petroleum product. By using the FBG, up to 10% of contamination can be easily detected [56]. Etched fiber Bragg grating (EFBG) has been used for this purpose. This is fabricated using the hydrogen loading technique. A solution of 20 ml of petrol and diesel with different adulteration is used for experimenting.

Figure 2.5 shows the experimental setup for this. The interrogator has four ports, and it acts as a source as well as the receiver. Each port is connected with a grating. The grating can be connected using a circulator, and the transmission spectrum can be monitored using a desktop. After performing the experiment, the center wavelength can be determined. This is the Bragg wavelength with respect to the air. After getting a reading of Bragg wavelength, we pour solutions with a different concentration on the disk in such a way that the grating must be fully dipped in the solution. After two minutes, we will get a shift in the center wavelength. This method measures the contamination in petroleum solutions. Various combinations of liquid with different

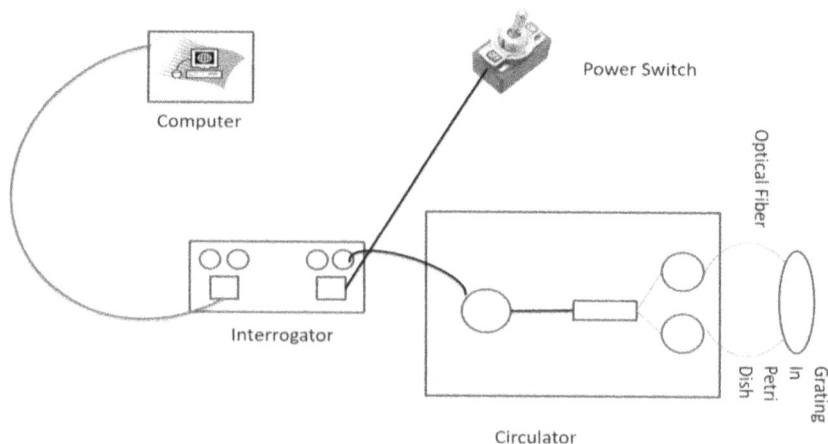

Figure 2.5 Experimental set up of FBG for fuel sensing.

concentration, behave as a binary liquid, and the resultant refractive index is given by Equation 2.14:

$$R.I. = \frac{n_1 V_1 + n_2 V_2}{V_1 + V_2} \qquad (2.14)$$

For Medical Devices: An optical sensor based on the polymer Bragg grating is very useful for biomedical industries because of their compatibility with biomedical applications, showing resistance in magnetic interference and avoiding any fragmentation when broken down. But, they are expensive [57, 58]. By the use of an environmental chamber having 30% humidity, thermal tests have been organized in biomedical industries. In another study, 7 ms polymer FBG was used for monitoring various human vital signs. An FBG was attached to the patient's chest for monitoring his or her respiratory system, and it could be analyzed by shifted wavelength. Similarly, an analysis of the heartbeat signal could be done. In the polymer optical fiber Bragg grating, wavelength shifting is 30 times (at least) longer than silica FBG (for both respiratory function and heartbeat monitoring) [59].

Liquid Sensing by Dual-optical Fiber Sensor: A liquid-sensing system with a cantilever, whose surface has uniform strength, is passed through the fiber Bragg grating (see Figure 2.6). A column buoy is fixed at one end of the cantilever which is dipped in the measuring liquid. When the level of measuring liquid changes, a force is applied on the end of the cantilever. The Bragg grating gets modified, due to strain or deformation, which is because of applied force. Hence, the Bragg wavelength shifts from the initial Bragg wavelength applied at one end of the cantilever beam. The shift in wavelength can be determined by Equation 2.15:

$$\Delta \lambda_B = \lambda_B \left(1 - P_e\right) KF \qquad (2.15)$$

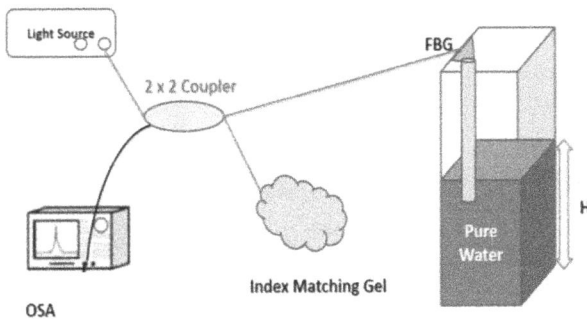

Figure 2.6 Liquid sensing through dual-optical fiber sensor.

where

λ_B: intial Bragg wavelength

$\Delta\lambda_B$: bragg wavelength shift(after applying the force)

K: strain sensitivity

P_e: strain optic coeffient

F: force

Thus, the measurement of liquid level can be performed by seeing the shift in Bragg wavelength.

Liquid-level Sensor Based on Tapered Chirped Fiber Grating: In this, the system has two clamps (moveable and fixed) and the tapered chirped grating is placed between them (see Figure 2.7). A clamp is connected with a column buoy which is partially dipped in a liquid tank. Now, a strain comes in the tapered chirped grating due to liquid-level variation causing a vertical pull by the column buoy. Here, variation in the liquid level applied on the vertical pull buoy results in axial strain. Thus, a shift in wavelength occurs [61].

Liquid Sensing Based on Archimedes' Law of Buoyancy: Liquid-level sensing (using optical fiber) based on Archimedes' law of buoyancy is versatile. One end of the FBG is fixed, whereas the other end is subjected to the mass suspended in the liquid (see Figure 2.8). According to Archimedes' law of buoyancy, "The Buoyant Force is an upward direction applied force when a body is at rest position in fluid, This Buoyant Force is equal to the weight of the fluid that the body displaces. The volume of the body is equal to the volume of fluid displaced when the body is completely submerged." Here, the total load F_T is given by the cylindrical mass, on the optical fiber when the liquid level (h) increases from the condition $h = 0$ (i.e., the liquid starts being in contact with the suspended mass) up to h_{max} (i.e., the maximum height allowed for water) [62].

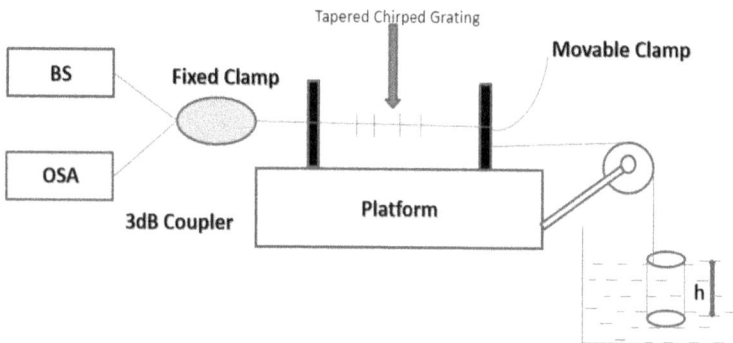

Figure 2.7 Liquid sensing through tapered chirped fiber grating.

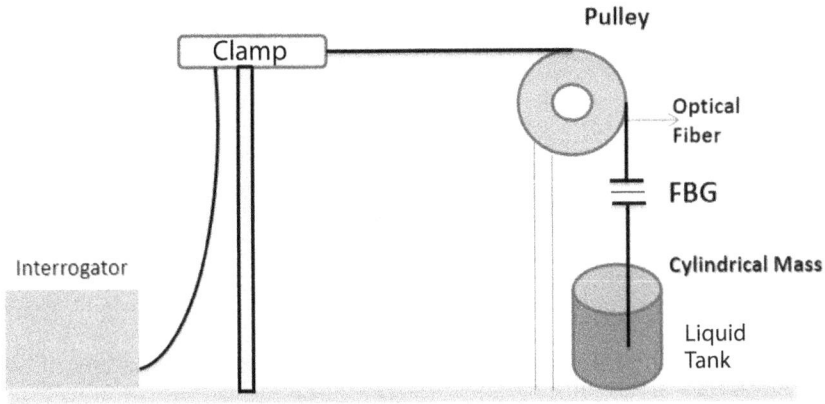

Figure 2.8 Schematic representation of the FBG liquid-level sensor based on Archimedes' law of buoyancy.

2.5 CONCLUSION

In this chapter, different grating structures and different shading for grating of the index were discussed for liquid-sensing applications. Here, uniform and apodization grating are used. In studies, it is clear that uniform grating is not as good for sensing applications when compared with cosine and raised cosine gratings, as both have fewer side lobes and reduced bandwidth. The FBG with structures is used for different liquid-sensing applications, such as the measurement of different contamination levels of fuel. We can easily measure up to 10% contamination using the above technique. Measurement of liquid is also done by the polymer fiber Bragg grating. Many other FBG-based structures for liquid-level sensing were also discussed.

REFERENCES

[1] K. Loizou and E. Koutroulis, "Water level sensing: State of the art review and performance evaluation of a low-cost measurement system", *Measurement*, vol. 89, pp. 204–214, 2016.

[2] B. W. Northway, N. H. Hancock, and T. Tran-Cong, "Liquid level sensors using thin walled cylinders vibrating in circumferential modes", *Meas. Sci. Technol.*, vol. 6, p. 85, 1995.

[3] F. N. Toth, G. C. M. Meijer, and M. van-der-Lee, "A planar capacitive precision gauge for liquid level and leakage detection", *IEEE Trans. Instrum. Meas.*, vol. 46, p. 644, 1997.

[4] A. Wang, M. F. Gunber, K. A. Murphy, and R. O. Claus, "Fiber-optic liquid-level sensor", *Sens. Actuators A*, vol. 35, p. 161, 1992.

[5] P. Raatikainen, I. Kassamakov, R. Kakanakov, and M. Luukkala, "Fiber-optic liquid-level sensor", *Sens. Actuators A*, vol. 58, p. 93, 1997.

[6] Kenneth O. Hill and Gerald Meltz, "Fiber bragg grating technology fundamentals and overview", *J. Light. Technol.*, vol. 15(8), pp. 1263–1276, 1997.

[7] G. Meltz, W. W. Morey, and W. H. Glenn, "Formation of bragg gratings in optical fibers by a transverse holographic method", *Opt. Lett.*, vol. 14(15), pp. 823–825, 1989.

[8] G. A. Ball, W. W. Morey, G. Hull-Allen, and C. Holton. "Low noise single frequency linear fibre laser", *Electron. Lett.*, vol. 29(18), pp. 1623–1625, 1993.

[9] G. A. Ball, W. W. Morey, and J. P. Waters, "Nd 3+ fibre laser utilising intra-core bragg reflectors", *Electron. Lett.*, vol. 26(21), pp. 1829–1830, 1990.

[10] William W. Morey, James R. Dunphy, and Gerald Meltz, "Multiplexing fiber bragg grating sensors", in *Fiber and Integrated Optics*, vol. 10 pp. 351–360. International Society for Optics and Photonics, 1992.

[11] G. Betta, L. Ippolito, A. Pietrosanto, and A. Scaglione, "Optical fiber-based technique for continuous-level sensing", *IEEE Trans. Instrum. Meas.*, vol. 44(3), pp. 686–689, 1995.

[12] W. Wang and F. Li, "Large-range liquid level sensor based on an optical fibre extrinsic Fabry–Perot interferometer", *Opt. Lasers Eng.*, vol. 52, pp. 201–205, 2014.

[13] K Spenner, M D Smgh, H Schult and H J Boehnel, "Expenmental mvestlgatlon of fiber optic hqmd level sensors and refractometers", *Proceeding Fuxt International Conference Optical Fiber Sensors*, London, UK, pp. 96–99, 1983.

[14] O. Fuentes, I. Del Villar, J.R. Vento, A.B. Socorro, E.E. Gallego, J.M. Corres, and I.R. Matias, "Increasing the Sensitivity of an Optic Level Sensor With a Wavelength and Phase Sensitive Single-Mode Multimode Single-Mode Fiber Structure", *IEEE Sens. J.*, vol. 17(17), pp. 5515–5522, 2017.

[15] Y. Jiang, W. Jiang, B. Jiang, A. Rauf, C. Qin, and J. Zhao, "Precise measurement of liquid-level by fiber loop ring-down technique incorporating an etched fiber", *Opt. Commun.*, vol. 351, pp. 30–34, 2015.

[16] G. Tsigaridas, D. Polyzos, A. Ioannou, M. Fakis, and P. Persephonis, "Theoretical and experimental study of refractive index sensors based on etched fiber Bragg grating", *Sens. Actuators, A*, vol. 209, pp. 9–15, 2014.

[17] M. Lomer, A. Quintela, M. López-Amo, J. Zubia, and J. M. López-Higuera, "A quasi-distributed level sensor based on a bent side-polished plastic optical fibre cable", *Meas. Sci. Technol.*, vol. 18(7), p. 2261, 2007.

[18] B. Yun, N. Chen, and Y. Cui, "Highly sensitive liquid-level sensor based on etched fibre Bragg grating", *IEEE Photonics Technol. Lett.*, vol. 19, pp. 1747–1749, 2007.

[19] P. Antunes, J. Dias, T. Paixão, E. Mesquita, H. Varum, and P. André, "Liquid level gauge based in plastic optical fiber", *Measurement*, vol. 66, pp. 238–243, 2015.

[20] F. N. Toth, G. C. M. Meijer, and M. van-der-Lee, "A planar capacitive precision gauge for liquid level and leakage detection", *IEEE Trans. Instrum. Meas.*, vol. 46, p. 644, 1997.

[21] A. Wang, M. F. Gunber, K. A. Murphy, and R. O. Claus, "Fiber-optic liquid-level sensor", *Sens. Actuators A*, vol. 35, p. 161, 1992.

[22] P. Raatikainen, I. Kassamakov, R. Kakanakov, and M. Luukkala, "Fiber-optic liquid-level sensor", *Sens. Actuators A*, vol. 58, p. 93, 1997.

[23] W. Wang and F. Li, "Large-range liquid level sensor based on an optical fibre extrinsic Fabry–Perot interferometer", *Opt. Lasers Eng.*, vol. 52, pp. 201–205, 2014.

[24] O. Fuentes, I. Del Villar, J.R. Vento, A.B. Socorro, E.E. Gallego, J.M. Corres, and I.R. Matias, "Increasing the sensitivity of an optic level sensor with a wavelength and phase sensitive single-mode multimode single-mode fiber structure", *IEEE Sens. J.*, vol. 17(17), pp. 5515–5522, 2017.

[25] Y. Jiang, W. Jiang, B. Jiang, A. Rauf, C. Qin, and J. Zhao, "Precise measurement of liquid-level by fiber loop ring-down technique incorporating an etched fiber", *Opt. Commun.*, vol. 351, pp. 30–34, 2015.

[26] G. Tsigaridas, D. Polyzos, A. Ioannou, M. Fakis, and P. Persephonis, "Theoretical and experimental study of refractive index sensors based on etched fiber Bragg grating", *Sens. Actuators, A*, vol. 209, pp. 9–15, 2014.

[27] P. Antunes, J. Dias, T. Paixão, E. Mesquita, H. Varum, and P. André, "Liquid level gauge based in plastic optical fiber", *Measurement*, vol. 66, pp. 238–243, 2015.

[28] B. Yun, N. Chen, and Y. Cui, "Highly sensitive liquid-level sensor based on etched fibre Bragg grating", *IEEE Photonics Technol. Lett.*, vol. 19, pp. 1747–1749, 2007.

[29] K.R. Sohn, and J.H. Shim, "Liquid-level monitoring sensor systems using fiber Bragg grating embedded in cantilever", *Sens. Actuators A*, vol. 152, pp. 248–251, 2009.

[30] T. Guo, Q.D. Zhao, Q.Y. Dou, H. Zhang, L.F. Xue, G.L. Huang, and X.Y. Dong, "Temperature-insensitive fibre Bragg grating liquid-level sensors based on bending cantilever beam", *IEEE Photonics Technol. Lett.*, vol. 17, pp. 2400–2402, 2005.

[31] C.W. Lai, Y.L. Lo, J.P. Yur, and C.H. Chuang, "Application of fiber Bragg grating level sensor and Fabry–Pérot pressure sensor to simultaneous measurement of liquid level and specific gravity", *IEEE Sens. J.* vol. 12, pp. 827–831, 2012.

[32] Q. Jiang, D. Hu, and M. Yang, "Simultaneous measurement of liquid level and surrounding refractive index using tilted fiber Bragg grating", *Sens. Actuators A Phys.*, vol. 170(1–2), pp. 62–65, 2011.

[33] C. B. Mou, K. M. Zhou, Z. J. Yan, H. Y. Fu, and L. Zhang, "Liquid level sensor based on an excessively tilted fiber grating", *Opt. Commun.*, vol. 305, pp. 271–275, 2013.

[34] G. Betta, A. Pietrosanto, and A. Scaglione, "A digital liquid level transducer based on optical fiber", *IEEE Trans. Instrum. Meas.*, vol. 45(2), pp. 551–555, 1996.

[35] M. Lomer, A. Quintela, M. López-Amo, J. Zubia, and J. M. López-Higuera, "A quasi-distributed level sensor based on a bent side-polished plastic optical fiber cable", *Meas. Sci. Technol.*, vol. 18(7), pp. 2261–2267, 2007.

[36] C. Zhao, L. Ye, X. Yu, and J. Ge, "Continuous fuel level sensor based on spiral side-emitting optical fiber", *J. Contr. Sci. Eng.*, vol. 2012, p. 267519, 2012.

[37] T. Imai, T. Komukai, and M. Nakazawa, "Dispersion tuning of a linearly chirped fiber Bragg grating without a center wavelength shift by applying a strain gradient", *IEEE Photonics Technol. Lett.*, vol. 10, pp. 845–847, 1998, doi: 10.1109/68.681505.

[38] K.O. Hill, F. Bilodeau, B. Malo, T. Kitagawa, S. Theriault, D.C. Johnson, J. Albert, and K. Takiguchi, "Chirped in-fiber Bragg gratings for compensation of optical-fiber dispersion", *Opt. Lett.*, vol. 19, pp. 1314–1316, 1994, doi: 10.1364/OL.19.001314.

[39] K.M. Feng, J.X. Chai, V. Grubsky, D.S. Starodubov, M.I. Hayee, S. Lee, X. Jiang, A.E. Willner, and J. Feinberg, "Dynamic dispersion compensation in a

10-Gb/s optical system using a novel voltage tuned nonlinearly chirped fiber Bragg grating", *IEEE Photonics Technol. Lett.*, vol. 11, pp. 373–375, 1999, doi: 10.1109/68.748240.

[40] S. Lee, R. Khosravani, J. Peng, V. Grubsky, D.S. Starodubov, A.E. Willner, and J. Feinberg, "Adjustable compensation of polarization mode dispersion using a high-birefringence nonlinearly chirped fiber Bragg grating", *IEEE Photonics Technol. Lett.*, vol. 11, pp. 1277–1279, 1999, doi: 10.1109/68.789716.

[41] J.X. Cai, K.M. Feng, A.E. Willner, V. Grubsky, D.S. Starodubov, and J. Feinberg, "Simultaneous tunable dispersion compensation of many WDM channels using a sampled nonlinearly chirped fiber Bragg grating", *IEEE Photonics Technol. Lett.*, vol. 11, pp. 1455–1457, 1999, doi: 10.1109/68.803077

[42] G. Palumbo, D. Tosi, A. Iadicicco, and S. Campopiano, "Analysis and design of Chirped fiber Bragg grating for temperature sensing for possible biomedical applications", *IEEE Photonics J.*, vol. 10, 2018, doi: 10.1109/JPHOT.2018.2829623

[43] A. Nand, D.J. Kitcher, S.A. Wade, T.B. Nguyen, G.W. Baxter, R. Jones, S.F. Collins, "Determination of the position of a localized heat source within a chirped fibre Bragg grating using a Fourier transform technique", *Meas. Sci. Technol.*, vol. 17, pp. 1436–1445, 2006, doi: 10.1088/0957-0233/17/6/023

[44] S. Yashiro, T. Okabe, N. Toyama, and N. Takeda, "Monitoring damage in holed CFRP laminates using embedded chirped FBG sensors", *Int. J. Solids Struct.*, vol. 44, pp. 603–613, 2007, doi: 10.1016/j.ijsolstr.2006.05.004.

[45] Dong XiaoWei, Liu WenKai, and Zhao RuiFeng, "Liquid-level sensor based on tapered chirped fiber grating", *Sci. China*, vol.56, no. 2, pp. 471–474, February 2013, doi: 10.1007/s11431-012-5095-z

[46] A. Othonos, "Fibre Bragg gratings", *Rev. Sci. Instrum.*, vol. 68, pp. 4309–4341, 1997.

[47] R. Nogueira, R. Oliveira, L. Bilro, and J. Heidarialamdarloo, "New advances in polymer fiber Bragg gratings", *Opt. Laser Technol.*, vol. 78, pp. 104–109, 2016.

[48] K. Peters, "Polymer optical fiber sensors—A review", *Smart Mater. Struct.*, vol. 20, no. 1, pp. 13002–13017, 2010.

[49] D. J. Webb, "Fiber Bragg grating sensors in polymer optical fibers", *Meas. Sci. Technol.*, vol. 26, no. 9, 2015, Art. no. 092004.

[50] M. C. J. Large, J. H. Moran, and L. Ye, "The role of viscoelastic properties in strain testing using microstructured polymer optical fibres (mPOF)", *Meas. Sci. Technol.*, vol. 20, p. 034014, 2009.

[51] M. Silva-Lopez, A. Fender, W. N. MacPherson, J. S. Barton, J. D. Jones, D. Zhao, H. Dobb, D. J. Webb, L. Zhang, and I. Bennion, "Strain and temperature sensitivity of a single-mode polymer optical fiber", *Opt. Lett.*, vol. 30, pp. 3129–3131, 2005.

[52] T. X. Wang, Y. H. Luo, G. D. Peng, and Q. J. Zhang, "High-sensitivity stress sensor based on Bragg grating in BDK-doped photosensitive polymer optical fiber", *Proc. SPIE*, vol. 8351, p. 83510M, 2012.

[53] C. A. F. Marques, A. Pospori, D. Sáez-Rodríguez, K. Nielsen, O. Bang, and D. J. Webb, "Aviation fuel gauging sensor utilizing multiple diaphragm sensors incorporating polymer optical fiber bragg gratings", *IEEE Sens. J.*, vol. 16, pp. 6122–6129, 2016.

[54] C. Broadway, R. Min, A. G. Leal-Junior, C. Marques, and C. Caucheteur, "Toward commercial polymer fiber bragg grating sensors: review and applications by christian broadway", *J. Light. Technol.*, vol. 37, no. 11, 01 June 2019, doi: 10.1109/JLT.2018.2885957

[55] G. D. Peng, Z. Xiong, and P. L. Chu, "Photosensitivity and gratings in dye-doped polymer optical fibers", *Opt. Fiber Technol.*, vol. 5, pp. 242–251, 1999.

[56] Sajal Agarwal, "A Dissertation Report on, Analysis and Characterization of Fiber Bragg Grating for Sensing Applications", June 2014.

[57] H.Y. Tam, C.-F.J. Pun, G.Y. Zhou, X. Cheng, and M.L.V. Tse, "Special structured polymer fibers for sensing applications", *Opt. Fiber Technol.*, vol. 16, pp. 357–366, 2010.

[58] P. Roriz, O. Frazão, A.B. Lobo-Ribeiro, J.L. Santos, J.A. Simões, "Review of fiber-optic pressure sensors for biomedical and biomechanical applications", *J. Biomed. Opt.*, vol. 18, p. 50903, 2013.

[59] Julien Bonefacino, "Ultra-fast polymer optical fibre Bragg grating inscription for medical devices", *Light Sci. Appl.*, vol. 7, p. 17161, 2018.

[60] Chih-Wei Lai, "Application of fiber bragg grating level sensor and fabry-pérot pressure sensor to simultaneous measurement of liquid level and specific gravity", *IEEE Sens. J.*, vol. 12, no. 4, April 2012, doi:10.1109/JSEN.2011.2161075

[61] Dong XiaoWei, "Liquid-level sensor based on tapered chirped fiber grating", *Sci. China Technol. Sci.*, vol. 56, no.2, pp. 471–474, February 2013, doi: 10.1007/s11431-012-5095-z

[62] M. Consales, "A fiber bragg grating liquid level sensor based on the Archimedes' law of buoyancy", *J. Light. Technol.*, doi: 10.1109/JLT.2018.2866130

Chapter 3

A Review of Multi-material, Multi-gate MOSFET Structures

Nagalakshmi Yarlagadda, Yogesh Kumar Verma and Manoj Singh Adhikari

Lovely Professional University, Punjab, India

Varun Mishra

Graphic Era (deemed to be a university), Uttarakhand, India

CONTENTS

ABBREVIATIONS

DGTFET	Double gate tunnel field effect transistor
DIBL	Drain induced barrier lowering
DMGAATFET	Dual material gate all around tunnel field effect transistor
FEDMGAA	Ferro electric dual material gate all around
GAA	Gate all around
GC-DMGJL	Graded channel dual material gate junction less
GIDL	Gate induced drain lowering
HEMT	High electron mobility transistor
HfO2	Hafnium oxide
JL DG MOSFET	Junction less double gate metal oxide semiconductor field effect transistor
JLDGTFET	Junction less Double gate Tunnel field effect transistor
MgZnO	Magnesium Zinc Oxide
MOSFET	Metal oxide semiconductor field effect transistor

DOI: 10.1201/9781003431138-3

RF   Radio Frequency
SCE   Short channel effect
SiO2   Silicon dioxide
SOI   Silicon on insulator
TCAD   Technology computer aided design
TFET   Tunnel field effect transistor
UG-DMGJL   Uniform channel dual material gate junction less
ZnO   Zinc oxide

3.1 INTRODUCTION

The importance of metal-oxide semiconductors (MOS) devices has considerably expanded. Therefore, large numbers of researchers have been working on MOS devices for the past few decades [1]. The complexity in fabrication of these devices has reduced with small modifications in electrical parameters, and scaling techniques increase the performance of the devices [2]. Serious problems have arisen with scaling MOS devices, and these include: high off-state current, drain-induced barrier lowering (DIBL) [3], low on-current, sub-threshold slope, more power consumption, more GIDL (i.e., gate-induced drain lowering) and high-power dissipation which degrades the devices' electrical competence. Several modifications in MOS devices are required to overcome these challenges. Gate current is controlled by introducing the multi-gate FinFET (field effect transistors), GAAFET (gate-all-around field effect transistors) and metal oxide semiconductor field effect transistor (MOSFET) with double gate [4]. Power dissipation minimization is required in the technology scaling, and therefore, the portable devices' battery life has been improved. The silicon on insulator (SOI) wafers are used in the structures of multi-gate MOSFETs and these are gate-all-around (GAA), triple-gate and double-gate MOSFETs. These structures have control on the subthreshold region gates and the process of less leakage with low power consumption in comparison with conventional MOSFETs [5, 6].

DIBL (drain-induced barrier lowering) with channel length decrement along with pinch-off raises the reliability problems associated with short channel effects (SCE), and also increasing drain voltage because of a hot-carrier effect [7]. Moreover, drain off-current increment and sub-threshold slope degradation are possible because of the increase in the gate voltage to control the drain current. If channel length is too short then, gate and drain terminals are very close to each other and bottleneck opens at high drain voltage which turns on the transistor in advance. MOS transistors ideal output characteristics are obtained when possible low value for DIBL then because of channel potential drain field effect, threshold voltage variations are reduced [8]. The equation (3.1) [9] represents the expression of DIBL.

$$\text{DIBL} = \frac{V_{th}^{dd} - V_{th}^{low}}{V_{dd} - V_{th}^{low}} \cdots \tag{3.1}$$

Beyond 100nm, the performance of the conventional MOSFET is maintained to the scaling trends, channel-length reduction causes different adverse effects. Because of microelectronic scaling of short channels and reduction in device electrical performance, multi-gate MOSFET, tri-gate MOSFET and double-gate MOSFET structures have been designed to reduce short channel effects. Many challenges were resolved with the double-gate MOSFET structure, such as junction capacitance and short-channel effects, and because of its low-power consumption and high-speed implementation it made a mark in MOS technology. A junction-less transistor is a widely used device for increasing packaging density [10]. For reverse-biased junction, the conventional MOSFET is turned off, [11]. In sub-nanometer technology, between the gate material and doped silicon, the work-function difference causes the depletion.

According to ON- and OFF-state performance, several advanced MOSFET structures are compared in this chapter. The MOSFET channel inversion operation before the region is called the subthreshold region. Reliable and required MOSFET performances are obtained by the deciding factor of subthreshold parameters [12].

3.1.1 ON-state Current

ON-state MOSFET is a state at which the threshold voltage of MOSFET is less than the gate voltage. In this state, current flow is defined as ON-state current, and it is represented as I_{ON}. From source, electrons are transferred toward the drain.

3.1.2 OFF-state Current

The MOSFET is in OFF-state, that is, no current flows between drain and source, When the gate voltage is less than threshold voltage, the flow of current is due to the presence of minority charge carriers between source and drain which is known as subthreshold current. The OFF-state MOSFET is a state at which the MOSFET V_{th} (threshold voltage) is greater than the gate voltage. In this state, current flow is defined as OFF-state current, which is because of minority charge carriers and is represented as I_{OFF}. Another name for the OFF-state current is subthreshold current.

3.1.3 Threshold Voltage

Channel inversion occurs when there is a minimum amount of voltage between gate and source, which is generally known as MOSFET threshold voltage (V_T). Gate-to-source voltage is minimum for nMOS transistor. Surface inversion is caused by the V_{gs} therefore, the conducting channel is established in between the drain and the source. There is no current flow for the condition $V_{gs} > V_{th}$ in between the source and the drain. High channel current in between the source and the drain through the minority charge carriers is required for the condition $V_{gs} > V_{th}$. But width of depletion region and surface potential remain constant as beyond the threshold voltage V_{gs} is increased [13].

3.1.4 Transconductance

The ratio between drain current variation and transistor gate voltage over a smalltime interval is called transconductance and is denoted with g_m. Required amplifier gain is obtained with transconductance with higher values [14]. The expression of g_m [9] is represented by equation (3.2).

$$g_m = \frac{2I_{ds}}{|V_P|}\left(1 - \frac{V_{gs}}{V_P}\right)\ldots \tag{3.2}$$

3.1.5 Stability Factor

MOS transistors two-port equivalent circuit parameters mainly influence the stability factor (k). In radio frequencies range (RF), transistors conditional stability is decided by this stability factor and it is expressed by equation (3.3) [15].

$$K = \frac{2\,\mathrm{Re}\left[Y_{11}\right]\mathrm{Re}\left[Y_{22}\right] + \mathrm{Re}\left[Y_{12}Y_{21}\right]}{\left[Y_{12}Y_{21}\right]}\ldots \tag{3.3}$$

Here, input and output admittance parameters are denoted as Y_{11} and Y_{22} at ports 1 and 2 respectively. Transfer admittances are denoted with Y_{12} and Y_{21}.

3.1.6 Subthreshold Slope (SS)

The gate terminal controls the drain current in the subthreshold region and the respective current is abruptly reduced. A suitable value of subthreshold slope (~60 mV/decade) is required to control the heating effect. The drain current is controlled by the gate terminal in the subthreshold region, and it is decreased. Subthreshold slope is given from the bulk and source voltages, voltage with drain and drain current plot slope. In short-channel devices, heating effects are controlled by selecting the subthreshold slope with a suitable value (approximately 60 mV/decade). The expression of subthreshold slope is represented by equation (3.4) [9].

$$SS_{th} = \ln(10)\frac{kT}{q}\left(1 + \frac{C_d}{C_{OX}}\right)\ldots \tag{3.4}$$

3.1.7 Junction Capacitance

In the MOSFET, junction capacitances are formed because of charge depletion between the substrate and source/drain. With respect to the source/grain
voltage, changes are attained in charged depletion. When the gate voltage is
more than the threshold voltage, the channel forms at the surface. In RF frequency range, transistor small signal analysis uses the junction capacitances
as deciding factors. New transistor structures and future scaling trends are
decided by the factors of ON- and OFF-state parameters of the MOSFET
[16]. Memory, digital circuit, biomedical applications and analog/RF applications are different applications which influence the MOSFET structure
design. The DC and AC performance parameters are calculated for performance analysis of MOSFET applications which are studied in this chapter.
Desired performance is achieved by using important circuit design analysis.

3.2 LITERATURE SURVEY

An 18nm, gate-length modified, junction-less SOI MOSFET study and analysis is presented by Vibhaas Saxena et al. [17]. Junction-less SOI transistors
are limited by the main challenges and low subthreshold slope, I_{on} to I_{off}
(on-current to off-current) ratio and high-leakage current. These challenges
are solved by introducing the slightly doped p-type silicon as a new window
inside the conventional, junction-less SOI MOSFET buried oxide region.
Less chip area and electrical performances are improved with the new optimizing windows which are below the gate length, channel area and modified SOI MOSFET. Junction-less BOX (buried oxide thickness) thickness is
analyzed.

Sentaurus technology computer aided design (TCAD) is used for the simulation. The equations of charge continuity are used for calculation of holes
and electron movement. Band analysis and drain current calculations are
used for the transport model of energy equalization. Referenced conditions
with self-heating condition combinations are considered, along with the hot
electron effects. Modified junction-less SOI transistors with different input
characteristics are also analyzed in this chapter. At buried oxide interface
and channel, depletion region formation is the main advantage of the
described method in order to obtain more benefits than the conventional
silicon on insulator junction less transistor (SOI-JLT). In this study, BOX
thickness reduction is used in reduction of leakage current.

The low-leakage pocket junction-less DGTFET (double gate tunnel field
effect transistor) is described by Suman Lata Tripathi et al. [18], along with
the biosensing cavity region. $Si_{0.7}Ge_{0.3}$ Narrow band gap material pocket
region with DGTFET shows band-to-band tunneling increment and makes
the threshold characteristics for achieving the digital and memory applications with high speed and low power. Atmospheric changes are effectively

detected in the junction less double gate field effect transistor (JLDGTFET) with cavity region, which automatically changes the threshold voltage and drain current.

Gate contact materials (Al, Pt, etc.) and the gate (SiO$_2$, HfO$_2$, etc.) are different oxide materials which are used in investigation of the described method. Because of gate influence, near the source region Si$_{0.7}$Ge$_{0.3}$ (energy band gap of <1 eV) pocket region with 5nm thickness is included for increasing the tunneling property of band-to-band. An oxide region made of SiO$_2$ (3.9) instead of high-K dielectric material HfO$_2$ (25) under Al/SiO$_2$ interface performance is compared, and Pt (5.7 eV) is used for the metal gate, which has a greater value of work function for achieving the high ON-state current. Figure 3.1 represents the cross-sectional view of double-gate MOSFET.

The cavity region with the pocket Si$_{0.7}$Ge$_{0.3}$ JLDGTFET ON/OFF performance is examined to improve the sensing capability for biomolecules that appear in the atmosphere. Therefore, if air present in the cavity dielectric constant is influenced, then overall performance is changed.Si$_{0.7}$Ge$_{0.3}$ JLDGTFET novel thin body pocket is simulated by using the 2D/3D visual TCAD tool.

In the analog domain, graded channel, dual-material gate junction-less MOSFET (GC-DMGJL MOSFET) is described for applications by Pathak et al. [19]. Uniform channel, dual-material gate junction cells (UC-DMGJL) MOSFET performance is evaluated with GC-DMGJL.

Short-channel effects reduction, high trans-conductance and drain current are the results of GC-DMGJL MOSFET. Near the channel drain region device, exists a high doping area $N_{gd} = 2.5 \times 10^{19}$ cm^{-3} and uniformly doped the remaining area of the device with $N_d = 2 \times 10^{19}$ cm^{-3}. $L_{M1} : L_{M2}$(nm) = 15 : 15 is the ratio of metal length. $W_{M1} : W_{M2}$(eV) = 5.353 : 4.8 is the metal work function ratio. 2 nm is the oxide thickness. W_{sp} = 10 nm is spacer length. T_{Si} = 10 nm is silicon thickness.

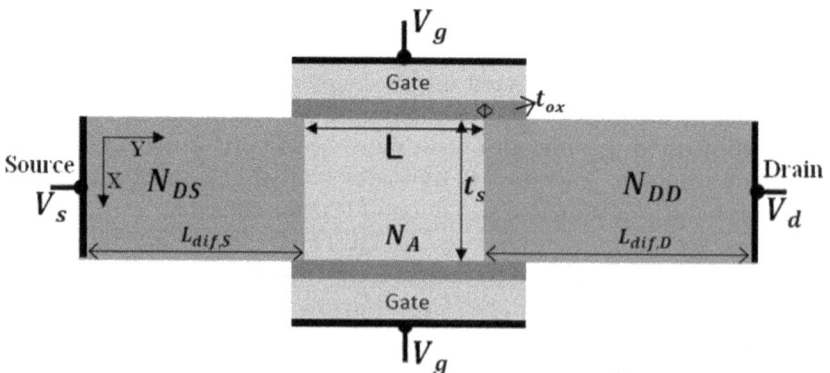

Figure 3.1 Cross-sectional view of double-gate MOSFET.

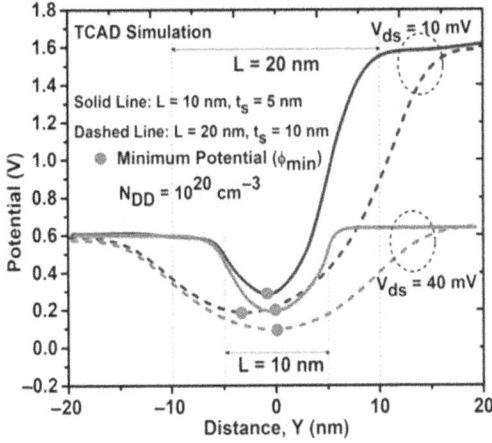

Figure 3.2 Calculation for the distribution of electric potential in the channel for different channel length at $V_{DS} = 10$ mV and 40 mV.

A surface-potential-based analysis of MgZnO/ZnO high electron mobility transistors (HEMT) is presented by Verma et al. [20]. The transistor structure with high electron mobility is designed and simulated in this paper. Simulation techniques are used to calculate the device parameters and the results demonstrate that this method is efficiently used by all for commercial circuit applications, with all reliability criteria.

Nitride and gallium arsenide-based devices have fewer drain currents as compared to the described method drain current. Fewer scattering effects are processed in the high electron mobility transistors (HEMT) than in the traditional MOSFETs. Figure 3.2 represents the calculation for the distribution of electric potential in the channel for different channel length.

Enhanced electrical performance with ferroelectric dual material gate all around-TFET (FEDMGAA-TFETs) structures is described by Varun Mishra et al. [21]. Drain current increased by the negative capacitance with the development of gate terminal internal positive feedback, which is noticeable by the ferroelectric material. The FEDMGAA-TFETs electrical characteristics are developed in this paper. Ferroelectric layer and ferroelectric material thickness changes are examined in the device performance. Ferroelectric layer relations with polarization and coercive field are very difficult. Ferroelectric layer thickness impact is investigated by the practical analysis of the device performance at polarization and fixed coercive field. The high thickness of ferroelectric layer does improve the drain current, which is observed from the results. The ferroelectric material thickness changes insignificantly alter the device OFF current.

Ferroelectric material uses the better contender as Si: HfO_2 in comparison with PZT and SBT as perovskite material, which gives the better scaling for nanometer range also. Switching ratio (I_{ON}/I_{OFF}) and ON current improvements are observed from the results. Therefore, low-voltage and energy-efficient applications utilize the described dual material gate all around-TFET (DMGAA-TFET).

Radiation and temperature, like extrinsic reliability issues on SiGe HBT, are introduced by Verma et al. [22]. Intrinsic and extrinsic are two types in SiGe HBT reliability issues which are analyzed in this paper. Inherent tradeoff between base resistance and DC current gain is the Si bipolar transistors fundamental limitation. A trade-off occurs because of the introduction of the injected electrons and holes back in the base and emitter respectively. . Therefore, currents of hole and electron both apply the same thermal push for a given thermal excitation and are then optimized with the higher supply of mobile electrons to the emitter, and the higher supply of mobile holes to the base. Hence, in base, ionized acceptor concentration is reduced, and current gain is increased, which results in the high base resistance. Figure 3.3 represents the calculation of gate capacitance with respect to gate voltage for L = 20nm and ts = 10nm.

For high-speed mode, at 77 K maximum cut off frequency as 155 GHz is observed and called the cryogenic temperature. High speed mode gain is maximum at 77 K as 25.5 dB. Therefore, it is clear that maximum gain value and maximum cut off frequency are obtained at cryogenic temperatures of SiGe HBT. In silicon transistor neutron radiation, the effect on transistor gain is also studied fully, because these effects influence the performance of the transistor gain.

In JL DG MOSFETs, two types are analyzed for gate underlap condition by Ajay et al. [23]. Two cases are considered for evaluation in this paper.

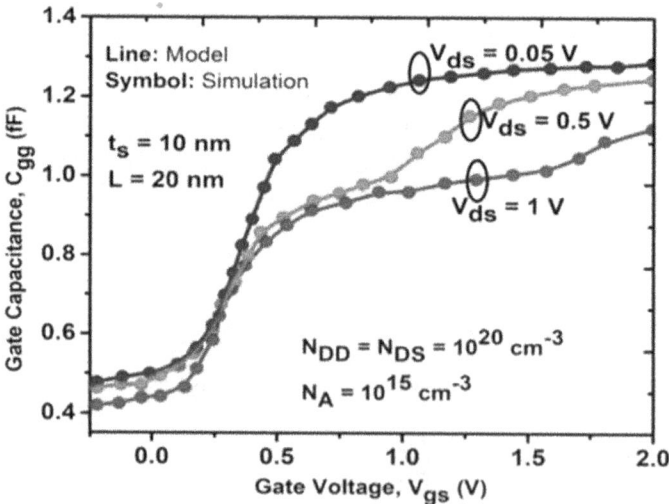

Figure 3.3 calculation of gate capacitance WRT gate voltage for L = 20nm and t_s = 10nm

The channel region of JL DG MOSFET source end portion has the under-lapped gate region, which is included in the first case. The channel region of JL DG MOSFET drain end portion has the underlapped gate region, which is included in the second case. Dielectric modulation techniques are used in detecting the biomolecules with these two types of structures. On JL DG MOSFET surface potential effect is produced by the charged biomolecules.

There is a movement for surface potential upwards because of positively charged biomolecules, and movement for surface potential downwards because of negatively charged biomolecules. 50nm as cavity length, 19nm as cavity thickness, 50nm as gate length, 10nm as gate oxide thickness, 20nm as channel thickness, source/drain and channel doping is $1 \times 10^{24} m^{-3}$, and 1 nm as oxide layer thickness in open cavity are the device parameters.

The reliability issues concerning junction less double gate (JLDG) MOSFETs are discussed by Abhinav et al. [9]. Thermal stability between 200 and 500K and gate misalignments are studied in this paper. The cur-rents in these structures are reduced with the misalignments in gate, then the performance of the JLDG MOSFETs. The MOSFET performance is also affected by the front and back gate alignments. Back gate shifting towards the source or drain side causes the effect of misalignment. Non-ideal effects are produced from the gate misalignments [24].

Device parameters dimensions are as follows: 1nm of front gate oxide thickness, 1nm of back gate thickness, 5 nm of silicon substrate thickness, $3 \times 10^{19} cm^{-3}$ is value of doping concentration N_d, 5.2 eV as gate work func-tion and 20 nm of channel length.

Junction less double gate (JLDG) MOSFET simulation and analytical sur-face potential modeling for ultra-low power analog/RF circuits are pre-sented by Nirmal Ch. Roy et al. [25]. Source, channel and drain are uniformly doped with the $N^+ - N^+ - N^+$ structure of N-channel junction-less double-gate (JL DG) transistor, Channel length and channel thickness, along with surface potential distribution of the described model, is derived. The chan-nel of the p-n junction of the described junction-less MOSFET does not have the same doping levels as the source/drain region. The ATLAS device simula-tor is used for the comparative numerical evaluation of the analytical model.

Model good approximation is provided by the ATLAS device simulator for comparative numerical evaluation of the analytical model. Higher immu-nity for SCEs is provided to the junction-less double-gate MOSFET as com-pared to the junction based double gate MOSFET, which is observed from the results. After comparative analysis, 17.08% of (I_{ON}/I_{OFF}) current ratio is increased, 4.52% of decreased amount of DIBL, and 1.61% of decreased subthreshold slope are the different parameters observed. Short-channel effects of DG MOSFET with junction is observed to be high when compared to JLDG MOSFET. Therefore, the (I_{ON}/I_{OFF}) ratio, subthreshold swing and DIBL are influenced by the doping concentration of JLDG MOSFET, which is observed from the results, similar to [26].

3.3 CONCLUSION

This chapter has provided an overview of multi material-based, multi-gate MOSFET structures. Different MOSFET structures are explored in this study with structural dimensions. Primarily, MOSFET structure modifications focus on reducing short-channel effects such as DIBL, hot electron effect biosensing cavity region with junction-less DGTFET, SOI transistor, junction-less SOI transistor, junction less double gate (JL DG) MOSFET, GC-DMGJL MOSFET, and transparent gate-recessed channel MOSFET. Using TCAD, RF performance investigations are included in this paper. Multi-gate junction-less MOSFETs provide improved individual outcomes to match future scaling trends while increasing MOS technology compatibility for any RF or IoT application as well as digital/analog applications.

REFERENCES

[1] Ming Qiao, Yong Chen, Dican Hou, Linrong He, Peipei Meng, Sen Zhang, Zhaoji Li, Bo Zhang, "Depletion MOS controlled current regulator diode based on bipolar carrier transport", *2021 33rd International Symposium on Power Semiconductor Devices and ICs (ISPSD)*, Year: 2021.

[2] Takashi Hamano, Keiichiro Urabe, Koji Eriguchi, "5 Model analysis for effects of spatial and energy profiles of plasma process-induced defects in Si substrate on MOS –Device performance", *2020 International Conference on Simulation of Semiconductor Processes and Devices (SISPAD)*, Year: 2020.

[3] Patrick Hofstetter, Robert W. Maier, Mark-M. Bakran, "Influence of the threshold voltage hysteresis and the drain induced barrier lowering on the dynamic transfer characteristic of SiC power MOSFETs", *2019 IEEE Applied Power Electronics Conference and Exposition (APEC)*, Year: 2019.

[4] Aanchal Garg, Yashvir Singh, "Nanoscale SiGe double gate MOSFET (GG-MOSFET) for analog/RF circuits", *2019 International Conference on Electrical, Electronics and Computer Engineering (UPCON)*, Year: 2019.

[5] Vadthiya Narendar, Shrey, Naresh Kumar Reddy, "Performance enhancement of multi-gate MOSFETs using gate dielectric engineering", *2018 International Conference on Computing, Power and Communication Technologies (GUCON)*, Year: 2018.

[6] Yu-Feng Hsieh, Si-Hua Chen Nan-Yow Chen, Wen-Jay Lee, Jyun-Hwei Tsai, Chun-Nan Chen, Meng-Hsueh Chiang, Darsen D. Lu, Kuo-Hsing Kao, "An FET with a source tunneling barrier showing suppressed short channel effect for low-power applications", *IEEE Transactions on Electron Devices*, Volume: 65, Issue: 3, Year: 2018.

[7] Zixuan Sun, Zhuoqing Yu, Runsheng Wang, Jiayang Zhang, Zhe Zhang, Peimin Lu, Ru Huang, "Investigation of DIBL degradation in nanoscale FinFETs under various hot carrier stresses", *2018 14th IEEE International Conference on Solid-State and Integrated Circuit Technology (ICSICT)*, Year: 2018.

[8] Gaspard Hiblot, "DIBL–Compensated extraction of the channel length modulation coefficient in MOSFETs", *IEEE Transactions on Electron Devices*, Volume: 65, Issue: 9, Year: 2018.

[9] Rai S. Abhinav, "Reliability analysis of junctionless double gate (JLDG) MOSFET for analog/RF circuits for high linearity applications", *Microelectronics Journal*, Year: 2017.

[10] Manish Gupta, Abhinav Kranti, "Raised source/drain germanium junctionless MOSFET for subthermal OFF-to-ON transition", *IEEE Transactions on Electron Devices*, Volume: 65, Issue: 6, Year: 2018.

[11] Dipanjan Sen, Bijit Banik, Swarnil Roy, "Power and delay analysis of junctionless double gate CMOS inverter in near and sub-threshold regime", *2018 IEEE Electron Devices Kolkata Conference (EDKCON)*, Year: 2018.

[12] Gennady I. Zebrev, Vasily V. Orlov, Alexander S. Bakerenkov, Vladislav A. Felitsyn, "Compact modeling of MOSFET I – V characteristics and simulation of dose-dependent drain currents", *IEEE Transactions on Nuclear Science*, Volume: 64, Issue: 8, Year: 2017.

[13] V. K. Mishra, R. K. Chauhan, "Efficient layout design of junctionless transistor based 6-T SRAM cell using SOI technology", *ECS Journal of Solid State Science and Technology*, Volume: 7, Year: 2018.

[14] Harshit Agarwal, Chetan Gupta, Sagnik Dey, Sourabh Khandelwal, Chenming Hu, Yogesh Singh Chauhan, "Anomalous Transconductance in Long Channel Halo Implanted MOSFETs: Analysis and Modeling", *IEEE Transactions on Electron Devices*, Volume: 64, Issue: 2, Year: 2017.

[15] Marjani, S. and Hosseini, S.E., 2015, May. Analysis of radio frequency and stability performance on double-gate extended source tunneling field-effect transistors. In *2015 23rd Iranian Conference on Electrical Engineering* (pp. 1042–1046). IEEE.

[16] Hussain Sayed, Ahmed Zurfi, Jing Zhang, "Design and experiments of a SiC power MOSFET bidirectional switching power pole", *2016 IEEE 25th International Symposium on Industrial Electronics (ISIE)*, Year: 2016.

[17] Vibhaas Saxena, Yash Gupta, Suresh Kumar, Nitu Rao and Vimal Mishra, "Study and analysis of modified junction-less SOI MOSFET at 18nm gate length", *2020 6th International Conference on Signal Processing and Communication (ICSC)*, Year: 2020.

[18] Suman Lata Tripathi, Raju Patel, Vimal Kumar Agrawal, "Low leakage pocket junction-less DGTFET with biosensing cavity region", *Turkish Journal of Electrical Engineering and Computer Sciences*, Volume: 27, Issue: 4, Year: 2019.

[19] V Patak, G. Saini, "A Graded channel dual-material gate junction less MOSFET for analog applications", *Procedia Computer Science*, Volume: 125, Year: 2018.

[20] Yogesh Kumar Verma, Santosh Kumar Gupta, Varun Mishra, Prateek Kishor Verma, "Surface potential-based analysis of MgZnO/ZnO high electron mobility transistors", *2018 IEEE International Students' Conference on Electrical, Electronics and Computer Science*, 2018.

[21] Varun Mishra, Yogesh Kumar Verma, Prateek Kishor Verma, Santosh Kumar Gupta, "Ferroelectric dual material gate all around TFET architecture for enhanced electrical performance", *2018 15th IEEE India Council International Conference (INDICON)*, Year: 2018.

[22] Yogesh Kumar Verma, Varun Mishra, Prateek Kishor Verma, Santosh Kumar Gupta, "Impact of extrinsic reliability issues including radiation and temperature on SiGe HBT", *2018 International Conference on Computational and Characterization Techniques in Engineering & Sciences (CCTES)*, Year: 2018.

[23] Ajay, "Reliability analysis of junctionless double gate (JLDG) MOSFET for analog/RF circuits for high linearity applications", *Microelectronics*, Year: 2017.

[24] A. Kumar, N. Guptha, R. Chaujar, "TCAD RF performance investigation of transparent gate recessed channel MOSFET", *Microelectronics*, Year: 2016.

[25] Nirmal Ch. Roy, Abhinav Gupta, Sanjeev Rai, "Analytical surface potential modeling and simulation of junction-less double gate (JLDG) MOSFET for ultra low-power analog/RF circuits", *Microelectronics Journal*, Year: 2015.

[26] A. Sarkar, K. Das, S. De, "Effect of gate engineering in double gate MOSFETs for analog/RF applications", *Microelectronics Journal*, Year: 2012.

Chapter 4

A Study of TFET-based Biosensors with Dual Material Double Gate structure for High Sensitivity and Cost-effective Biomedical Applications

Kavindra Kumar Kavi and R.A. Mishra

Motilal Nehru National Institute of Technology Allahabad,
Uttar Pradesh, India

CONTENTS

ABBREVIATIONS

BBT	Band to band tunneling
BGN	Band gap narrowing
BJT	Bipolar junction transistor
BOD	Biochemical oxygen demand
DMDGDM	Dual material double gate dielectric modulated
FET	Field effect transistor
IL	Interleukin
IUPAC	International Union of Pure and Applied Chemistry
MOSFET	Metal oxide semiconductor FET

DOI: 10.1201/9781003431138-4

SRH	Shockley-Read-Hall
TFET	Tunnel field effect transistor
TOC	Total organic carbon
UTI	Urinary tract infection

4.1 INTRODUCTION

Earlier detection means that doctors have more time to treat the patients, and also to treat before the disease becomes more serious.

The major applications of biosensors are:

1. **Medical Diagnostic Field** – Glucose biosensors are in use in the health-care industry for diagnosis of diabetes mellitus. Biosensors can also be used for detection of urinary tract infection (UTI) and detection of human interleukin (IL)-10 antigen. Furthermore, they are being used for the quantitative measurement of cardiac markers for predicting cardiac arrests and also the accurate detection of multiple cancer markers [1–3].
2. **Food Industry** – Biosensors are extensively used in authenticity, quality and safety monitoring. To name a few specific applications: they are used for the monitoring of the ageing of beer in breweries, monitoring of the fermentation process, the detection of pathogens in food (most commonly as fecal contamination which is detected by the presence of E. coli) and the detection of pesticides in wines and juices. Not only that, but the monitoring of food quality parameters like the appearance of the food, its taste, smell, even the nutritional value, freshness, flavor, texture and so forth are carried out using biosensors [4–9].
3. **Environmental Monitoring** – Biosensors have use in environmental pollution monitoring. Analytes which have been measured are insecticides, herbicides, heavy metals and BOD (biochemical oxygen demand) among others [10–12].
4. **Hazardous Chemical Monitoring in Industries** – Similar to the above, industries also need to detect pollutants, BOD sensors, and TOC (total organic carbon) monitors among others [11, 12].
5. **Military Applications** – We can utilize biosensors for military applications for the purpose of keeping us safe in the event biological attacks. They can help us to detect and identify the threatening microorganisms which can be used as bio-warfare agents along with chemical toxins. For this application we need devices that are highly sensitive and selective [13].

Biosensors are instruments that make use of a biological recognition component that is kept in close proximity to a transducer. A biosensor, according to International Union of Pure and Applied Chemistry (IUPAC), is a device that may transform a physical or biological event into a quantifiable signal, typically an electrical one. The transduction stage is a critical stage as it converts

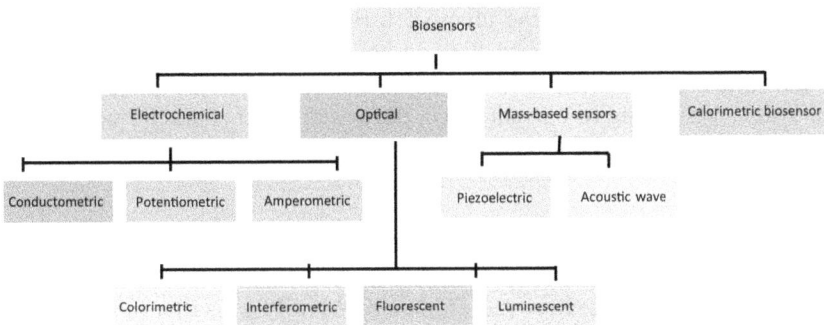

Figure 4.1 Types of biosensors.

the physiochemical reaction into a measurable electrical signal for further processing. This needs to be done quickly and should be extremely sensitive [14].

4.1.1 Types of Biosensors

Among the numerous varieties of biosensors available (see Figure 4.1), electrochemical biosensors are the most popular. This is because one type of electrochemical biosensors, the FET-(field effect transistor) based biosensors, have lower cost fabrication and offer superior performance, which includes label-free detection, small size leading to on-chip integration, rapid detection, reliable performance, superior selectivity and reusability [15]. We will focus on FET-based biosensors next.

4.1.2 FET Biosensors

As the name suggests, the field effect transistor has flow of current in the semiconductor material that is controlled by an applied electric field. The MOSFET (metal oxide semiconductor FET) is the most well-known and commonly utilized FET device used today (see Figure 4.2). The application

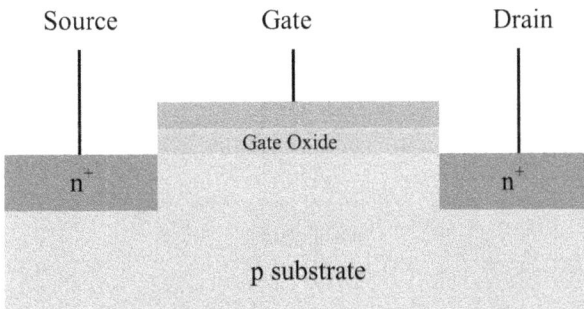

Figure 4.2 Simple MOSFET structure.

of gate voltage controls the channel formation between source and the drain. This affects the current flowing between drain and source. Unlike a bipolar junction transistor (BJT), FETs are unipolar devices (either electron or hole contributing to current). FET devices are also characterized by high input impedance [16].

4.2 TUNNEL FIELD EFFECT TRANSISTORS (TFETs)

The point of difference between TFETs and MOSFETs is that in a TFET, the source and drain have an opposite type of doping (Figure 4.3).

4.2.1 Quantum Tunneling

In the simplest words, quantum tunnelling is the phenomenon whereby a particle can pass through a potential barrier, even when it lacks the necessary energy to do so. This transmission probability (P_t) is given as follows:

$$P_t = \left\{ \frac{16}{3 + \dfrac{U_0}{E}} \right\} e^{-2k_2 a} \tag{4.1}$$

where,

$$k_2 = \frac{\sqrt{2m(U_0 - E)}}{\hbar} \tag{4.2}$$

In the Equations 4.1 and 4.2, U_0 = height of energy barrier, E = energy of the particle, a = tunneling width and m = mass of the particle. We can observe that as tunneling width decreases, the tunneling probability increases exponentially.

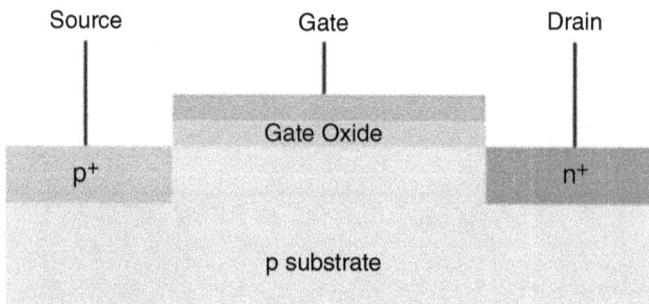

Figure 4.3 Simple TFET structure.

Additionally, the likelihood of tunnelling increases as $U_0 - E$ decreases if the barrier height U_0 is lowered or the particle's energy is raised. The probability of tunneling also rises as the particle's mass decreases. [17].

4.2.2 Subthreshold Swing

The rate at which the drain current rises as the gate voltage rises is known as the subthreshold slope and it measures this change in gate voltage in millivolts per decade (mV/decade). Now, let's see why MOSFET is not capable of giving low SS value [18].

For a MOSFET,

$$SS = \ln(10)\frac{kT}{q}\left(1 + \frac{C_d}{C_{ox}}\right) \tag{4.3}$$

where,

C_d = capacitance of the depletion region
C_{ox} = capacitance of gate oxide
$\frac{kT}{q}$ = thermal voltage.

For minimizing SS, we make $\frac{C_d}{C_{ox}} = 0$. Then we get $SS_{min} = \ln(10)\frac{kT}{q}$ which at room temperature comes out to be 60 mV/dec. This is the minimum theoretical limit of SS of a MOSFET device. Since TFETs don't rely on thermionic emission, they can achieve much lower SS than this.

4.2.3 Ambipolar Current

Despite the advantage of better SS, TFET still suffers from problems. These include, extremely low ON current and existence of ambipolar current. The methods adopted for mitigating these are deployed within the proposed device structure.

We can describe ambipolar current after going through the TFET energy band diagram and working principle in the next section.

4.3 DUAL MATERIAL DOUBLE GATE CAVITY INSERTED BIOSENSOR

It can be seen from the Figure 4.4 structure that we have two set of gates (top and bottom). This is called double gate structure and the benefit of using this scheme is that it helps to improve ON current (which we have earlier described as being one of the disadvantages of TFET) and also gives

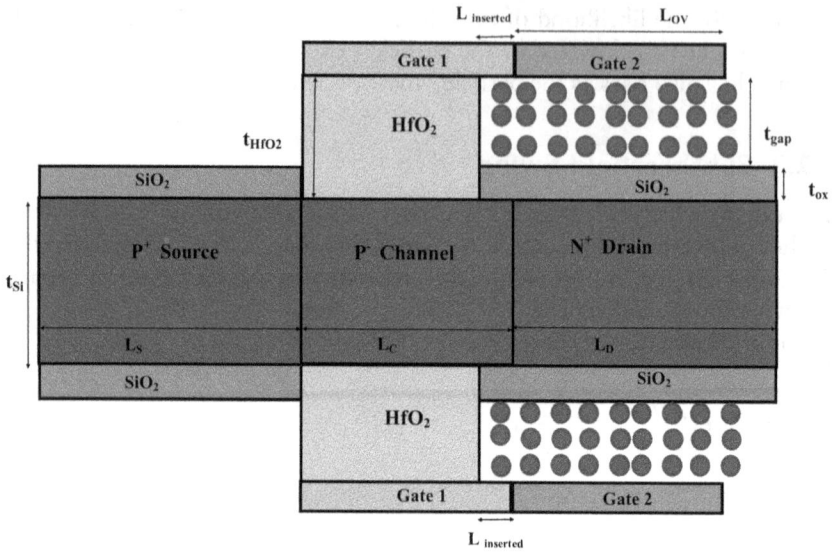

Figure 4.4 Proposed dual material double gate cavity inserted biosensor structure.

better gate control over the device operation. Also, we use dual material gates [19]. The channel-drain junction's barrier width is widened by the gate overlap on the drain side having greater work function, which reduces ambipolar current. One of the advantages of using the dielectric modulated nanocavity based structure is that it can be used to detect both neutral and varying dielectric constant which affects ambipolar current. Considering the decrease in the ambipolar current of the device, will improve in coupling capacitance and the tunneling width of the channel-drain region. The sensitivity of the biosensor is improved due to the tuned dielectric value of charged biomolecules that are trapped under the gate overlap on drain which forms a nano cavity.

Using dual material gate has its own advantages, which can be seen in Figure 4.5 above. As shown, we see that higher work function of gate 2 decreases ambipolar current even further. But as seen in the graphs, we realize that increasing work function gives only a small reduction in ambipolar drain current. For this reason, we choose a work function of 5.2 which belongs to the metal nickel. This simulation was carried out in Silvaco ATLAS software.

In ATLAS, for simulating the device performance, the BBT Kane model was used along with Shockley-Read-Hall (SRH), Auger recombination, Fermi Dirac, band gap narrowing (BGN) and field dependent mobility models [20, 21].

The device specifications are given in Table 4.1. The device is made of a 50nm silicon channel. It has a 10nm thick HfO_2 over the channel as

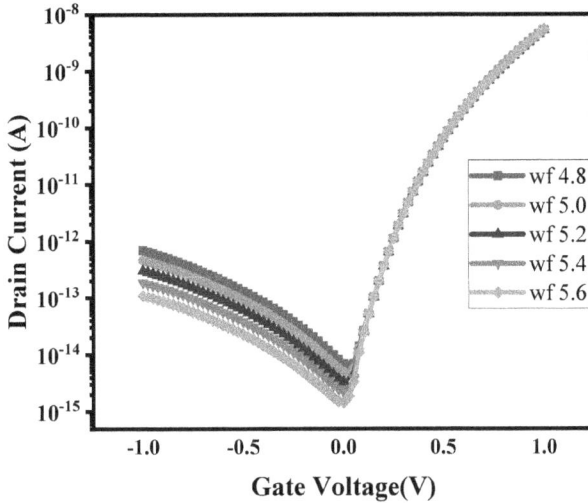

Figure 4.5 Variation in drain current with work function of gate 2.

Table 4.1 Device parameters and specifications used for simulation

Parameter	Symbol	Specification
Channel length (nm)	L_C	50
Drain length (nm)	L_D	100
Source length (nm)	L_S	100
Silicon thickness (nm)	t_{Si}	10
Cavity thickness (nm)	t_{gap}	9
Channel doping (cm^{-3})	N_A	10^{17}
Drain doping (cm^{-3})	N_D	10^{19}
Source doping (cm-^{3})	N_A	10^{20}
HfO$_2$ thickness (nm)	t_{HfO2}	10
SiO$_2$ thickness (nm)	t_{ox}	1
Work Function, Gate 1 (eV)	Φ_{M1}	4.8
Work Function, Gate 2 (eV)	Φ_{M2}	5.2
Length of cavity inserted (nm)	$L_{inserted}$	5

dielectric. The nanocavity is formed by the overlapping gate over the drain end. The cavity inserted portion is present over the channel. Biomolecules captured in the nanocavity are modeled as a dielectric material for the purpose of simulation. By varying its dielectric constant, we can model different biomolecules.

4.4 RESULTS AND DISCUSSION

4.4.1 Ambipolar Current Variation with Biomolecule Position

The length of cavity was divided into three regions with L_1, L_2 and L_3 lengths. From these, we define regions R_1, R_2 and R_3 as follows:-

R_1 = 0 to L_1, R_2 = L_1 to L_2 and R_3 = L_2 to L_3. Here 0 is taken as start of the nanocavity.

These are shown in Figure 4.4.

Therefore, having much more portion of cavity over the channel reduces the ambipolar current further (see Figure 4.6). This can be observed in the following section.

4.4.2 Variation of Ambipolar Current with Variation in $L_{inserted}$

We selected $L_{inserted}$ of 5nm as it gave better sensitivity as compared to reference dual material gate structure.

When a biomolecule is placed in the nanocavity, a reduction in the ambipolar current of the device is observed. As we change the dielectric value of biomolecules, the ambipolar current decreases further. This is utilized as the

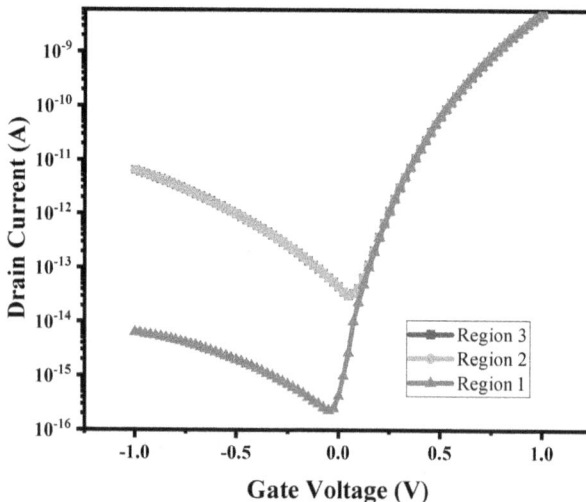

Figure 4.6 Variation in ambipolar current based on the regions it is filling in the nanocavity.

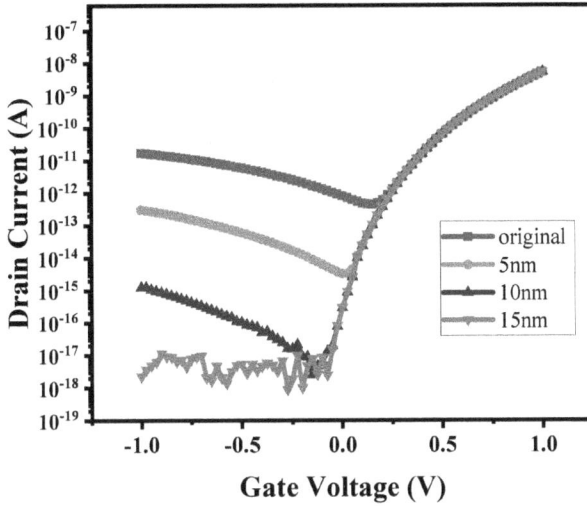

Figure 4.7 Variation in ambipolar current with the length of cavity inserted inside the channel.

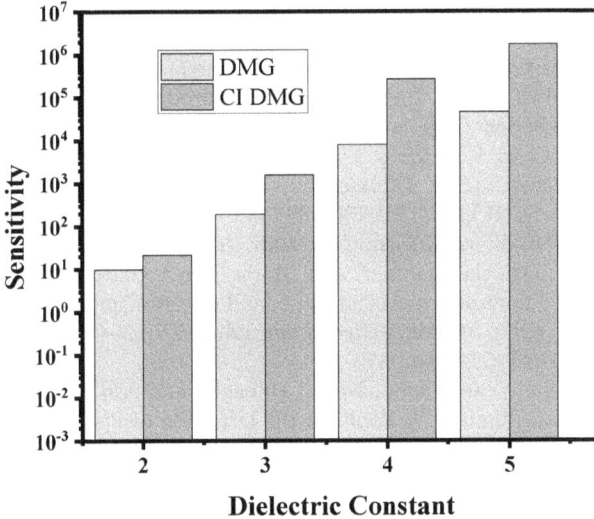

Figure 4.8 Sensitivity comparison between dual material gate [22] and proposed device for different dielectric constant biomolecules in cavity.

sensing phenomenon for biomolecule and, hence, we find the sensitivity using ambipolar current (see Figures 4.7 and 4.8). Mathematically, it is defined as:-

$$S = I_{DS}(\text{air}) / I_{DS}(\text{dielectric}) \tag{4.4}$$

4.5 CONCLUSION

In this chapter we have discussed how the TFET, DMDG structure is used to improve gate control and on current, and to reduce ambipolar current. We note that as the biomolecule's nanocavity's dielectric constant rises, correspondingly the ambipolar current decreases. This widens the channel-drain junction's tunneling barrier, which reduces the ambipolar current. We propose a cavity inserted structure. Finally, we completed a comparison between a dual material gate structure [22] and a proposed device, and showed that a proposed device has a higher sensitivity and, since gate 2 work function is chosen as zinc which is cheaper compared to the metal platinum in [22], we can conclude that it is cost-effective.

REFERENCES

1. Rogers, K.R., and J.N. Lin. 1992. "Biosensors for Environmental Monitoring." *Biosensors and Bioelectronics* 7 (5): 317–21. https://doi.org/10.1016/0956-5663(92)85026-7
2. Ercole, C., M. Del Gallo, L. Mosiello, S. Baccella, and A. Lepidi. 2003. "Escherichia Coli Detection in Vegetable Food by a Potentiometric Biosensor." *Sensors and Actuators B: Chemical* 91 (1): 163–68. https://doi.org/10.1016/S0925-4005(03)00083-2
3. Alì, G., and G. Frosali, 2005. "Quantum Hydrodynamic Models for the Two-Band Kane System." *Nuovo Cimento B* 120 (12): 1279.
4. Boucart, K., and A.M. Ionescu. 2007. "Double-Gate Tunnel FET with High-κ Gate Dielectric." *IEEE Transactions on Electron Devices* 54 (7): 1725–33. https://doi.org/10.1109/TED.2007.899389
5. Scognamiglio, Viviana, Gianni Pezzotti, Ittalo Pezzotti, Juan Cano, Katia Buonasera, Daniela Giannini, and Maria Teresa Giardi. 2010. "Biosensors for Effective Environmental and Agrifood Protection and Commercialization: From Research to Market." *Microchimica Acta* 170 (3–4): 215–25. https://doi.org/10.1007/s00604-010-0313-5
6. Arora, Pooja, Annu Sindhu, Neeraj Dilbaghi, and Ashok Chaudhury. 2011. "Biosensors as Innovative Tools for the Detection of Food Borne Pathogens." *Biosensors and Bioelectronics* 28 (1): 1–12. https://doi.org/10.1016/j.bios.2011.06.002
7. Lee, Michael, Nadia Zine, Abdellatif Baraket, Miguel Zabala, Francesca Campabadal, Raffaele Caruso, Maria Giovanna Trivella, Nicole Jaffrezic-Renault, and Abdelhamid Errachid. 2012. "A Novel Biosensor Based on Hafnium Oxide: Application for Early Stage Detection of Human Interleukin-10." *Sensors and Actuators B: Chemical* 175 (December): 201–7. https://doi.org/10.1016/j.snb.2012.04.090
8. Chen, Yi Wei, Maozi Liu, Tetsuya Kaneko, and Paul C. McIntyre. 2010. "Atomic Layer Deposited Hafnium Oxide Gate Dielectrics for Charge-Based Biosensors." *Electrochemical and Solid-State Letters* 13 (3): G29. https://doi.org/10.1149/1.3280224

9. Scognamiglio, V., F. Arduini, G. Palleschi, and G. Rea 2014. "Bio Sensing Technology for Sustainable Food Safety." *Trends Anal Chem.* 62: 1–10.

10. Ghasemi-Varnamkhasti, Mahdi, María Luz Rodríguez-Méndez, Seyed Saeid Mohtasebi, Constantin Apetrei, Jesus Lozano, Hojat Ahmadi, Seyed Hadi Razavi, and Jose Antonio de Saja 2012. "Monitoring the Aging of Beers Using a Bioelectronic Tongue." *Food Control* 25 (1): 216–24. https://doi.org/10.1016/j.foodcont.2011.10.020

11. Mishra, Rupesh K., Rocio B. Dominguez, Sunil Bhand, Roberto Muñoz, and Jean-Louis Marty. 2012. "A Novel Automated Flow-Based Biosensor for the Determination of Organophosphate Pesticides in Milk." *Biosensors and Bioelectronics* 32 (1): 56–61. https://doi.org/10.1016/j.bios.2011.11.028

12. Yan, Chen, Feng Dong, Bi Chun-Yuan, Zhu Si-Rong, and Shi Jian-Guo. 2014. "Recent Progress of Commercially Available Biosensors in China and Their Applications in Fermentation Processes." *Journal of Northeast Agricultural University (English Edition)* 21 (4): 73–85. https://doi.org/10.1016/s1006-8104(15)30023-4

13. Ghorbanpour, M., P. Bhargava, A. Varma, and D.K. Choudhary. 2021. *Biogenic Nano-Particles and Their Use in Agro Ecosystems.* Singapore: Springer Verlag.

14. Justino, Celine, Armando Duarte, and Teresa Rocha-Santos. 2017. "Recent Progress in Biosensors for Environmental Monitoring: A Review." *Sensors* 17 (12): 2918. https://doi.org/10.3390/s17122918

15. Mehrotra, Parikha. 2016. "Biosensors and Their Applications – A Review." *Journal of Oral Biology and Craniofacial Research* 6 (2): 153–59. https://doi.org/10.1016/j.jobcr.2015.12.002

16. Sarkar, D., and K. Banerjee. 2012. "Fundamental Limitations of Conventional-FET Biosensors: Quantum-mechanical-tunneling to the Rescue," in *IEEE 70th Device Research Conference.*

17. Abdi, Dawit Burusie, and M. Jagadesh Kumar. 2015. "Dielectric Modulated Overlapping Gate-on-Drain Tunnel-FET as a Label-Free Biosensor." *Superlattices and Microstructures* 86 (October): 198–202. https://doi.org/10.1016/j.spmi.2015.07.052

18. Anand, Sunny, and R.K. Sarin. 2016. "An Analysis on Ambipolar Reduction Techniques for Charge Plasma Based Tunnel Field Effect Transistors." *Journal of Nanoelectronics and Optoelectronics* 11 (4): 543–50. https://doi.org/10.1166/jno.2016.1922

19. Reddy, N. Nagendra, and Deepak Kumar Panda. 2020. "Simulation Study of Dielectric Modulated Dual Material Gate TFET Based Biosensor by Considering Ambipolar Conduction." *Silicon*, October. https://doi.org/10.1007/s12633-020-00784-9

20. Reddy, N. Nagendra, and Deepak Kumar Panda. 2020. "A Comprehensive Review on Tunnel Field-Effect Transistor (TFET) Based Biosensors: Recent Advances and Future Prospects on Device Structure and Sensitivity." *Silicon*, August. https://doi.org/10.1007/s12633-020-00657-1

21. Mamidala Jagadesh Kumar, Rajat Vishnoi, and Pratyush Pandey. 2017. *Tunnel Field-Effect Transistors (TFET): Modelling and Simulations.* Hoboken: Wiley.

22. Kavi, K.K., K. Kiroula, M. Kumar, A. Dwivedi, and R.A. Mishra. 2022. "Performance Evaluation of Dual Material Double Gate TFET based Biosensor." *7th Students' Conference on Engineering & Systems-2022.*

Chapter 5

Investigation of Domino Buffer Circuit in Biomedical Applications

Amit Kumar Pandey
Rajkiya Engineering College, Uttar Pradesh, India

Tarun Kumar Gupta
Maulana Azad National Institute of Technology Bhopal,
Madhya Pradesh, India

Shipra Upadhyay
Atria Institute of Technology, Karnataka, India

Vikas Patel
Rajkiya Engineering College, Uttar Pradesh, India

CONTENTS

ABBREVIATIONS

CMOS   Complementary metal oxide semiconductor
HSPICE   H(Hewlett)-Simulation Program with Integrated Circuit Emphasis
NMOS   N-channel metal oxide semiconductor
PMOS   P-channel metal oxide semiconductor

5.1 INTRODUCTION

Realization of complex gates using a static complementary metal oxide field effect transistor (CMOS) method requires a large area. It consists of a large stack of P-channel metal oxide semiconductor (PMOS) and N-channel metal oxide semiconductor (NMOS) transistors in the pull-up (PUN) and pull

DOI: 10.1201/9781003431138-5

down (PDN) networks respectively [1]. Parasitic capacitance at dynamic node and output node increases delay when using this method. The use of domino logic to realize a complicated gate lowers area and delay. It is employed in high-performance circuits, for example multiplexors [2, 3] and comparators [4, 5]. It is made up of a clocked PMOS precharge transistor, an NMOS footer transistor, and a PDN. Domino logic comprises two phases: precharge and evaluation [5].

A buffer circuit is required to connect a high impedance source to a low impedance load without signal distortion. It forwards the output of the domino circuit to the next level [6]. Toggling the output state in a static CMOS logic circuit dissipates power [7, 8]. This circuit costs power, owing to unnecessary duplicate transition at output and dynamic nodes. This duplicate transition problem consumes more power than static CMOS. To address this issue, various methods are offered, in survey. Static transition pulse domino logic [9] and single phase domino logic [10] remove unnecessary transition at both output and dynamic nodes, making it operate similarly to a static CMOS circuit. The use of limited switch dynamic logic (LSDL) [11, 12], true single phase clock domino logic (TSPC) [13, 14], and pseudo dynamic buffer (PDB) [15] avoids duplicate transition solely at output node. The dynamic power consumption of a domino circuit is the amount of power consumed all through capacitance charging and discharging. By lowering the power supply, dynamic power consumption is reduced, but the delay increases. Another method for lowering dynamic power consumption is to reduce capacitance; however this is a challenging operation because its value is governed by the circuit layout. Lower the circuit's transition activity to reduce dynamic power consumption.

In this study, a transition-aware approach is given that avoids duplicate transition at output and dynamic nodes while maintaining a circuit's static CMOS behavior. The pull up transistor is governed by a trigger pulse generator. When a clock and its inverting delayed clock are both high, the pull up transistor activates. Using this strategy, it is possible to propagate precharge pulse to dynamic node while avoiding precharge pulse to output node. This chapter is structured as follows. Section 5.2 discusses previous methods. Section 5.3 explains new circuits. Section 5.4 contains simulation findings, while Section 5.5 contains the conclusion.

5.2 SURVEY WORK

Figure 5.1 shows conventional footless domino logic. If input is held high, then this circuit operates in two operational phases. Transistor T1 is turned ON during the precharge phase. A dynamic node is first charged to a high voltage and then discharged. A dynamic node is drained to low voltage during evaluation, while the output is charged to high voltage. A dynamic node

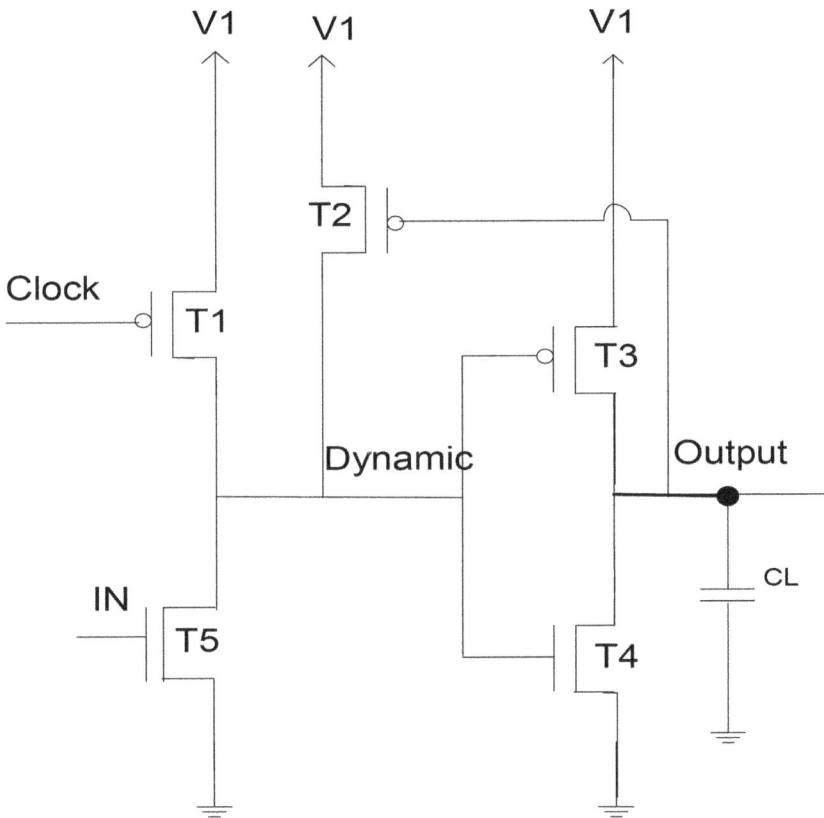

Figure 5.1 Schematic of conventional footless. This is also known as a standard footless circuit.

maintains a high level of performance in both working phases when the input is kept low. To make the circuit stable, precharge pulse propagation is required at dynamic node, but inhibited at output node. This duplicate transition at output and dynamic nodes consumes more power.

The problem of duplicate transition at both output and dynamic nodes is solved by SP-Domino [10]. As illustrated in Figure 5.2, SP-Domino is analogous to clock delayed domino [16]. The latest input does not appear before the delayed clock's rising edge. Because the dynamic node's PUN and PDN occur during the evaluation phase, the gate has a single phase. Transistor T1 is a pull up and keeper transistor. At the beginning of the evaluation cycle, the pulse generator generates signal P, which activates T1. When both transistors T1 and T10 are turned ON at the same time, during the duration of pulse P, a small amount of conflict current flows between them. The T1 charges dynamic node to high voltage when transistor T10 shuts off at the beginning of the evaluation phase. If the dynamic node at the end of the

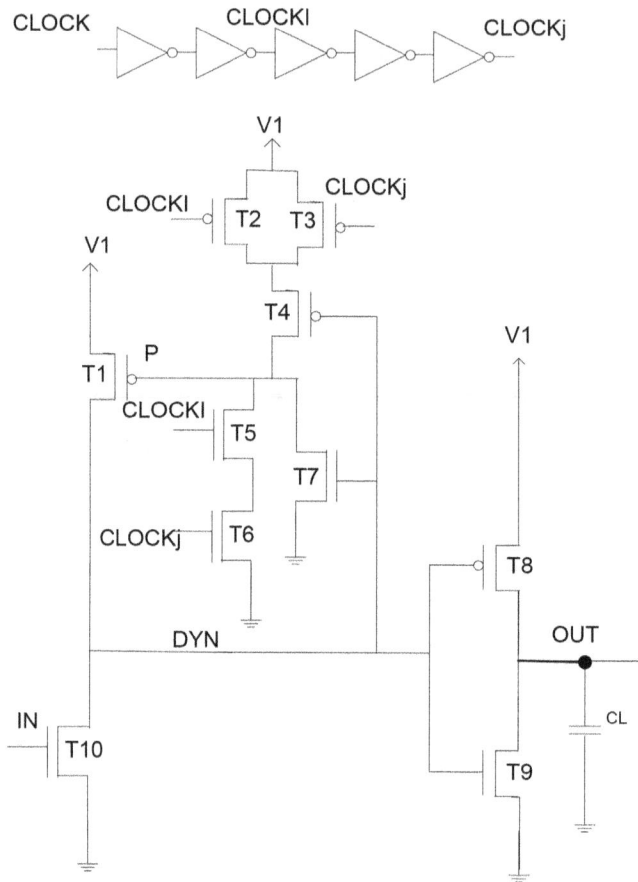

Figure 5.2 Schematic of SP-Domino. This figure also includes the triggering network.

pulse signal P has a low value, T7 is deactivated, and P is pulled high by transistor T4. The dynamic node's charging action begins when P returns to low voltage.

Another method for reducing duplicate transition at both output and dynamic nodes is static switching pulse domino (SSPD) [9]. The SSPD utilizes separate transistors T1 and T2, which are never both activated at the same time. The SSPD approach makes use of a conditional pulse generator (CPG). T1 activates only after dynamic node has been discharged or held low in the preceding evaluation cycle, and keeper T2 shuts off. T1 is turned off by CPG if dynamic node is not discharged. Transistor T8 is ON, and the keeper is providing conflict current. CPG generates two additional clock phases, $CCLK_d$ and $CCLK_i$, internally. Their actions are influenced by clock signal (CLK) and dynamic node.

5.3 NEW WORK

The designed buffer circuit is illustrated in Figure 5.3. Figure 5.4 demonstrates the timing intervals of clocks. It uses independent transistors T1 and T2 for pull up and keeper respectively. Trigger pulse generator (TPG) governs T1. The function of the TPG is to generate a brief duration low trigger pulse T at commencement of a clock high. The TPG is made up of two input NAND gates and inverting delays, where CLOCK is clock and CLKi is clock delayed inverting signal.

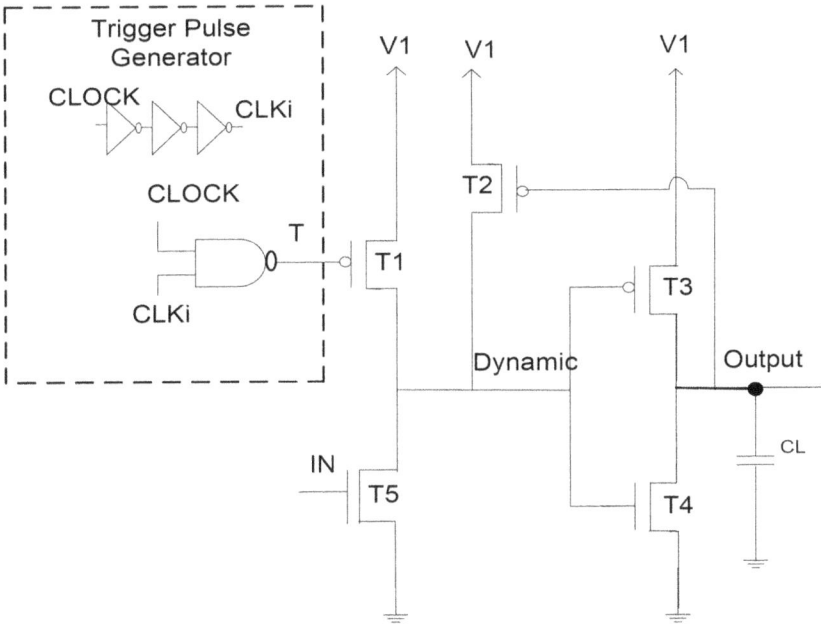

Figure 5.3 Schematic of new work. This figure includes trigger pulse generator.

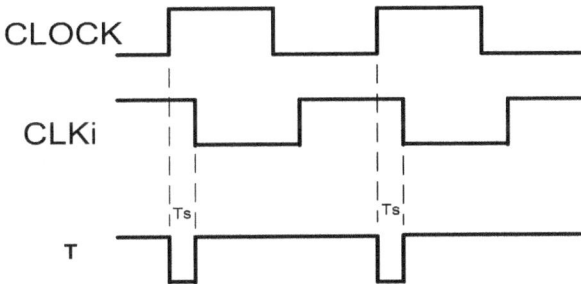

Figure 5.4 Timing intervals of the clocks. This clock pulses are applied to transistor T1.

Using this strategy, it is possible to propagate precharge pulse to the dynamic node while avoiding precharge pulse to the output node. Working is described by looking at the input logic. When the clock is set to zero, the dynamic node retains its previous value regardless of the inputs.

Situation 1: When input is high, T5 activates. CLOCK is high at the beginning of clock high, and delayed clock CLKi is high for a brief interval of time Ts. In the time interval T, the output of NAND output is low. When T1 and T5 are activated, they supply conflict current to the PDN. Following the time delay Ts, the trigger pulse generator output T raises high, and T1 deactivates. As a result, no additional conflict current flows to the PDN, and the dynamic node is still at logic low.

Situation 2: If input is low, CLOCK is high at beginning of clock, and CLKi is high at end of clock. When the trigger pulse is low, then T1 is activated, and the dynamic node is set to logic high. For the remainder of the clock high, time T is high, T1 goes OFF, and the dynamic node logic remains high. This buffer circuit is used in the prediction of neurotransmitters, EEG, stress, strain and exhaustion.

5.4 EXPERIMENT RESULTS

The new circuit and other available circuits, for example SP-Domino and conventional footless domino circuits, are modelled on 180 nm models using the H(Hewlett)-Simulation Program with Integrated Circuit Emphasis (HSPICE) tool [17]. All circuits operate at 200 MHz with a 50% duty cycle (clock period of 5 ns) and a 1.8 V supply voltage. To allow for a fair comparison, all of the circuits are of identical size. The worst-case delay is calculated from input node to output node. When the input voltage is high, power consumption is calculated.

Table 5.1 summarizes the power savings for several functions of the new circuit against the conventional circuit. The input frequency, clock frequency and load capacitance were all set to 50 MHz, 200 MHz, and 100fF, respectively, for this comparison. Table 5.1 reveals how increasing the fan-in of OR gates saves more power. Likewise, increasing the fan-in of AND gates reduces power usage.

Table 5.2 shows a power comparison of new and available circuits with a clock frequency of 200 MHz and varying load capacitance. For higher load capacitances, our new circuit reduces power consumption when compared to available circuits. In comparison to typical footless domino, SSPD, and SP-Domino approaches, this new circuit reduces power consumption by 3.1, 1.5 and 1.1 for capacitance 500fF. Our new circuit has less latency than the SP-Domino and SSPD circuits, although slightly more than the traditional footless domino circuit. as demonstrated in Table 5.3. As demonstrated in Table 5.4, our suggested circuit provides a better PDP and a lower saving at larger load capacitance than current circuits.

Table 5.1 Power-saving logic functions in 0.18 m

Function	Conventional circuit (in μW)	New circuit (in μW)	Power saved by new circuit (in %)
A	393.96	78.34	80.16
A + B	391.33	77.87	80.10
A.B	263.86	78.85	70.11
A + B + C	400.14	78.30	80.43
A.B.C	200.82	79.46	60.43
A + B + C + D	402.45	78.61	80.52
A.B.C.D	178.47	81.17	54.33
A.B + C.D	382.93	79.04	79.35

Notes: Clock Frequency = 200MHz, V_{DD} = 1.8 V, load capacitance = 100fF, and Input Frequency = 50MHz.

Table 5.2 Power consumption (μW) of new circuit versus available circuits

Load capacitance (fF)	Conventional domino	SP-Domino	SSPD	New circuit
100	394.95	113.31	95.49	78.34
200	416.25	129.64	114.69	97.42
300	449.84	146.04	134.19	116.73
400	462.72	162.74	154.16	136.28
500	480.85	178.32	172.86	155.09

Table 5.3 Delay (ps) of new circuit versus available circuits

Load capacitance (fF)	Conventional domino	SP-Domino	SSPD	New circuit
100	182.35	375.11	307.82	240.91
200	322.45	490.07	458.68	375.29
300	465.85	608.44	606.44	507.24
400	589.19	729.89	753.86	637.53
500	738.75	856.17	902.36	775.90

Table 5.4 Power delay product (fJ) of new circuit versus available circuits

Load capacitance (fF)	Conventional domino	SP-Domino	SSPD	New circuit
100	72.01	42.50	29.39	18.87
200	134.21	63.53	52.60	36.56
300	209.55	88.85	81.39	59.21
400	272.62	118.78	116.21	86.88
500	355.22	152.67	155.98	120.33

5.5 CONCLUSION

This paper introduces a new work circuit. The new circuit includes a trigger pulse generator that governs the circuit's pull up transistor. This technology reduces duplicate transition at output and dynamic nodes, which minimizes dynamic power consumption. It stops the dynamic node from receiving evaluation pulse and the output node from receiving the precharge pulse. HSPICE is used to simulate the new circuit as well as available circuits such as conventional footless domino, SSPD, and SP-Domino in 0.18 m technology. The suggested structure's performance is compared to that of existing circuits at various clock frequencies, stress conditions and temperatures. When compared to conventional circuits, our new circuit consumes less power. This buffer circuit is used in the prediction of neurotransmitters, EEG, stress, strain and exhaustion.

REFERENCES

[1] A. K. Pandey, T. K. Gupta, A. Gupta, and D. Pandey, "Keeper effect on nano scale silicon domino logic transistors", *Silicon*, Springer, vol. 25, pp. 6769–6776, 2021.

[2] Z. Liu, and V. Kursun, "Leakage biased PMOS sleep switch dynamic circuits", *IEEE Transactions on Circuits and Systems*, vol. 53, no. 10, pp. 1093–1097, 2006.

[3] H. Mahmoodi, and K. Roy, "Diode-footed domino: A leakage-tolerant high fan-in dynamic circuits design style", *IEEE Transactions on Circuits and Systems*, vol. 51, no. 3, pp. 495–503, 2004.

[4] K. J. Nowka, and T. Galambos, "Circuit design techniques for a gigahertz integer microprocessor", *IEEE International Conference on Computer Design*, pp. 11–16, 1998.

[5] A. Amirabadi, A. A. Kusha, Y. Mortazavi, and M. Nourani, "Clock delayed domino logic with efficient variable threshold voltage keeper", *IEEE Transactions on Very Large Scale Integration (VLSI) Systems*, vol. 15, no. 2, pp. 125–134, 2007.

[6] R. H. Krambeck, C. M. Lee, and H. Law, "High-speed compact circuits with CMOS", *IEEE Transactions on Journal of Solid State Circuits*, vol. 17, no. 3, pp. 614–619, 1982.

[7] S. Garg, and T. K. Gupta, "Very low power domino logic circuits using carbon nanotube field effect transistor technology", *Journal of Nanoelectronics and Optoelectronics*, vol. 14, no. 1, pp. 19–32, 2019.

[8] S. Garg, and T. K. Gupta, "Low power domino logic circuits in deep-submicron technology using CMOS", *Engineering Science and Technology, an International Journal*, vol. 21, no. 4, pp. 625–638, 2018.

[9] R. Singh, G. Moon, M. Kim, J. Park, W. Y. Shin, and S. Kim, "Static-switching pulse domino: A switching-aware design technique for wide fan-in dynamic multiplexers", *Integratiom, The VLSI Journal*, vol. 45, pp. 253–262, 2012.

[10] J. A. Charbel, and A. B. Magdy, "Single-phase SP-domino: A limited-switching dynamic circuit technique for low-power wide fan-in logic gates", *IEEE Transactions on Circuits and Systems*, vol. 55, pp. 141–145, 2008.

[11] S. Jayakumaran, C. N. Hung, J. N. Kevin, K. Robert, and B. Brown, "Controlled-load limited switch dynamic logic circuit", *IEEE Conference on Computer Society*, pp. 1–6, 2005.

[12] A. K. Pandey, R. A. Mishra, and R. K. Nagaria, "Low power dynamic buffer circuits", *International Journal of VLSI Design & Communication Systems (VLSICS), AIRCC Publication*, vol. 3, no. 5, pp. 53–65, 2012.

[13] F. Tang, and A. Bermak, "Low power TSPC-based domino logic circuit design with 2/3 clock load", *Transactions on Energy Procedia*, vol. 14, pp. 1168–1174, 2012.

[14] Y. J. Ren, I. Karlsson, and C. Svensson, "A true single-phase clock dynamic CMOS circuit technique", *IEEE Transactions on Solid-State Circuits*, vol. 22, pp. 899–901, 1987.

[15] T. Fang, B. Amine, and G. Zhouye, "Low power dynamic logic circuit design using a pseudo dynamic buffer", *Integration, the VLSI Journal*, vol. 45, pp. 395–404, 2012.

[16] G. Wei, and C. Sechen, "Clock-delayed domino for dynamic circuit design", *IEEE Transactions on Very Large Integration (VLSI) Systems*, vol. 8, no. 4, pp. 425–430, 2000.

[17] Berkeley Predictive Technology Model (BPTM), http://www.device.eecs.berkeley.edu/wptm/download.htm

Chapter 6

A Novel Digitally Controllable Variant of Extra-X Second Generation Current Conveyor and Its Filter Application Suitable for Biomedical Signal Processing

Bhartendu Chaturvedi and Jitendra Mohan
Jaypee Institute of Information Technology, Noida, Uttar Pradesh, India

Jitender
Ajay Kumar Garg Engineering College, Ghaziabad, India

CONTENTS

ABBREVIATIONS

ABB	Active building block
APF	All pass filter
CM	Current mode
CMOS	Complementary metal oxide semiconductor
DC-EXCCII	Digitally controllable extra-X second generation current conveyor
DCCB	Digital current controlling block
DCW	Digital control word
DCWC	Digital control word circuitry
DPCCII	Digitally programmable second generation current conveyor
DPCFA	Digitally programmable current feedback amplifier
DPDVCC	Digitally programmable differential voltage current conveyor
EXCCII	Extra-X second generation current conveyor
GCAPF	Gain controllable all pass filter
PSPICE	Personal simulation program with integrated circuit emphasis

DOI: 10.1201/9781003431138-6

6.1 INTRODUCTION

Current mode (CM) circuits have garnered more recognition in recent times compared to voltage mode circuits. The simple reason for this is the wide range of benefits offered by the current mode operation, such as: high bandwidth support, superior dynamic range and ability to operate at smaller supply voltages among others [1–4]. In 1968, the current conveyor was proposed by Sedra and Smith as the first ever active building block (ABB) which supports CM operation [5, 6]. Since then, a number of versatile current conveyor structures have emerged [7–16]. It is well recognized that these CM ABBs have the feature of unity current gain. However, there might be some applications in which output current controllability is an essential requirement. The conventional complementary metal oxide semiconductor (CMOS) structures of the ABBs would not help the cause in such scenarios. Therefore, the presence of a current controlling mechanism could prove to be beneficial. There are some current conveyor structures like the digitally programmable second generation current conveyor (DPCCII) [17], the digitally programmable differential voltage current conveyor (DPDVCC) [18] and the digitally programmable current feedback amplifier (DPCFA) [19] among others, which inherit the output current controllability feature. However, this highly desirable feature is not present in most of the prominently utilized ABBs of recent times. The EXCCII [14] is one such ABB which is extensively featuring in numerous signal processing applications at this time [20–27].

This chapter explores the idea of incorporating the current controllability feature in the standard EXCCII design. To show the usefulness of the idea, a gain controllable APF (GCAPF) configuration is also presented in the chapter. Both digitally controllable extra-X second generation current conveyor (DC-EXCCII) and GCAPF operate at small supply voltages of ±1 V and consume very little power. The inclusion of the digital current controlling block (DCCB) may additionally help in achieving the tunability of the frequency response of the designed application. The potential to operate in power constrained environments marks the suitability of DC-EXCCII and the designed GCAPF for signal processing applications in biomedical domain [28, 29].

6.2 PROPOSED DC-EXCCII

In the traditional EXCCII structure [14], a digital control word circuitry (DCWC) [30] is incorporated to realize its digitally controlled variant, that is, DC-EXCCII. The symbol of DC-EXCCII is shown in Figure 6.1. The CMOS configuration of DC-EXCCII depicting the merger of EXCCII and the CMOS based DCWC is shown in Figure 6.2. Transistors M_{12}-M_{19}, M_{26}-M_{33} are used to realize the additionally incorporated DCWC. Here, the 4-bit digital control word (DCW) "$C_0 C_1 C_2 C_3$" controls the gain of current transfer from X_2 to Z_2 port.

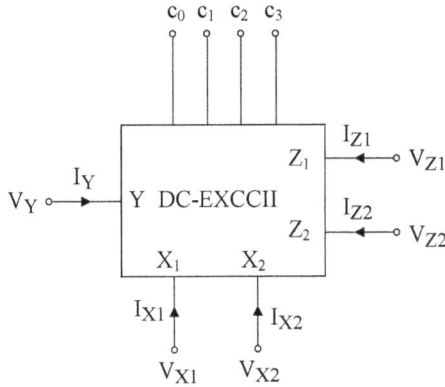

Figure 6.1 DC-EXCCII's symbolic representation.

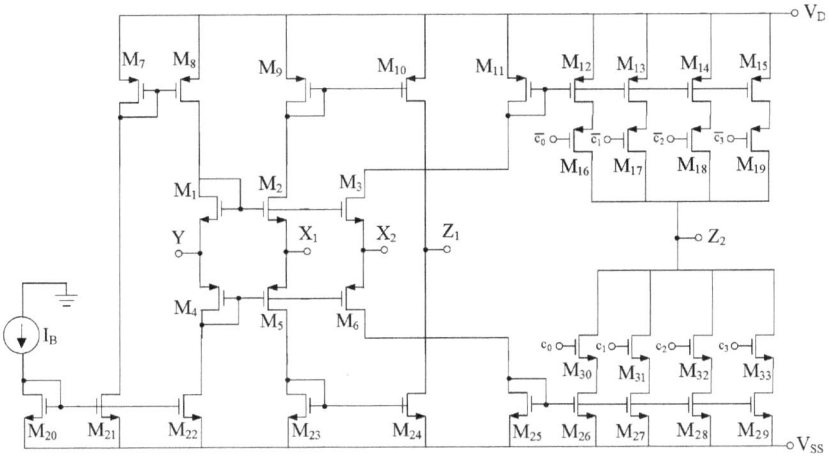

Figure 6.2 CMOS structure of proposed DC-EXCCII.

The DCWC has four branches which can be activated or deactivated by varying its 4-bits, that is, "$C_0 C_1 C_2 C_3$". The number of activated branches determines the current transfer gain (α_{Z2}) from X_2 to Z_2 port. Table 6.1 summarizes the realized current transfer gain values depending on the applied DCW values. It is worth mentioning that using an additional DCCB section for Z_1 stage will facilitate the current gain programmability from X_1 to Z_1 terminal as well. The equation describing the port relations of DC-EXCCII is expressed in Equation 6.1.

$$
\begin{bmatrix}
I_Y \\
V_{X1} \\
V_{X2} \\
I_{Z1} \\
I_{Z2}
\end{bmatrix}
=
\begin{bmatrix}
0 & 0 & 0 \\
1 & 0 & 0 \\
1 & 0 & 0 \\
0 & 1 & 0 \\
0 & 0 & \alpha_{Z2}
\end{bmatrix}
\begin{bmatrix}
V_Y \\
I_{X1} \\
I_{X2}
\end{bmatrix}
\tag{6.1}
$$

Table 6.1 Current control behavior of DC-EXCCII.

S. no.	4-bit DCW ($C_0C_1C_2C_3$)	Activation status of DCWC branches (Bi)				Input and output current relationship
		B_1 $M_{12}, M_{16},$ M_{26}, M_{30}	B_2 $M_{13}, M_{17},$ M_{27}, M_{31}	B_3 $M_{14}, M_{18},$ M_{28}, M_{32}	B_4 $M_{15}, M_{19},$ M_{29}, M_{33}	
1	1000	Activated	Deactivated	Deactivated	Deactivated	$I_{z2}= I_{x2}$, i.e. $\alpha_{z2}=1$
2	1100	Activated	Activated	Deactivated	Deactivated	$I_{z2}= 2I_{x2}$ i.e., $\alpha_{z2}=2$
3	1110	Activated	Activated	Activated	Deactivated	$I_{z2}= 3I_{x2}$, i.e. $\alpha_{z2}=3$
4	1111	Activated	Activated	Activated	Activated	$I_{z2}= 4I_{x2}$, i.e. $\alpha_{z2}=4$

6.3 DC-EXCCII'S VERIFICATION

DC-EXCCII's performance verification is done by carrying out personal simulation program with integrated circuit emphasis (PSPICE) simulations. For this purpose 180nm CMOS parameters are employed. The transistors' aspect ratios used for CMOS realization of DC-EXCCII are provided in Table 6.2. Bias current, I_B is chosen as 30 µA and supply voltages are ± 1V in magnitude. Proposed DC-EXCCII is first verified for unity gain current transfer from X_2 to Z_2 (DCW = "1000"). For unity gain setting, the voltage and current conveying relations are identical to the conventional EXCCII. This fact is supported by the simulation results obtained through various analyses during the simulations. Figures 6.3 and 6.4 show the linearity relationships for the DC voltage and current transfers, respectively. DC-EXCCII shows linearity from –400mV to 400mV and –200µA to 200µA for voltage and current transfers, respectively. Time domain waveforms obtained by performing transient analysis also justify the desired voltage and current transfer relationships.

Table 6.2 MOS transistors W/L ratios for DC-EXCCII's CMOS structure

MOS transistors	$W(\mu m)/L(\mu m)$
M_1–M_3, M_{20}–M_{33}	2.16/0.18
M_4–M_6	5.76/0.18
M_7–M_{19}	3.6/0.18

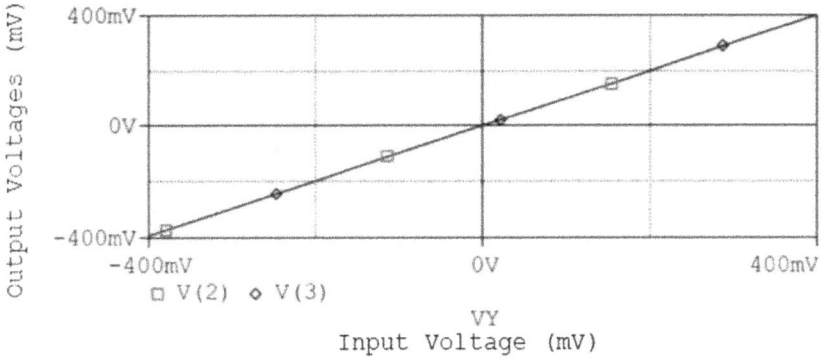

Figure 6.3 DC-EXCCII's voltage conveying action for unity gain.

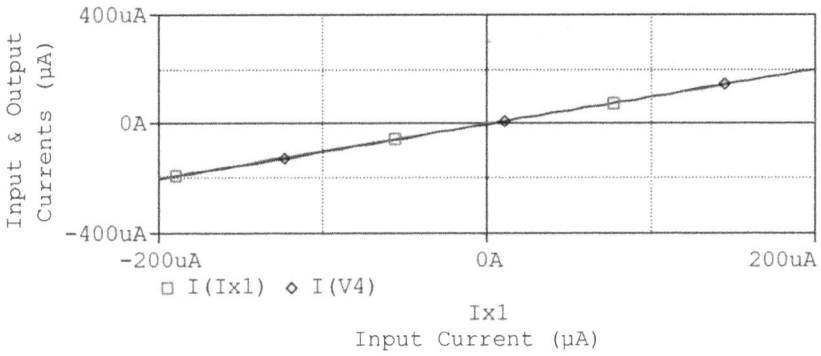

(a)

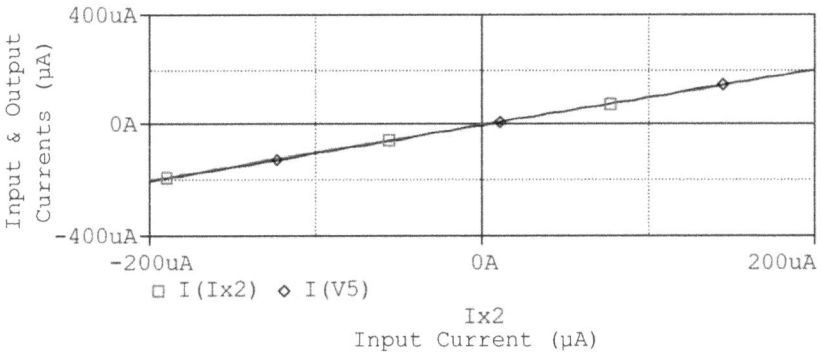

(b)

Figure 6.4 DC-EXCCII's current conveying action for unity gain a) X_1 to Z_1 b) X_2 to Z_2.

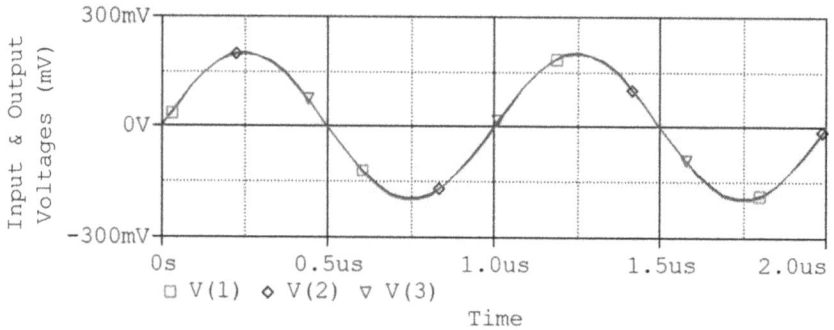

Figure 6.5 DC-EXCCII time domain voltage waveforms for unity gain.

Figure 6.5 shows the voltage conveying action between Y and X ports. Identically, Figure 6.6 depicts the current conveying action between X and Z ports. An estimate of the operating bandwidth of DC-EXCCII is obtained by performing AC analysis.

Figures 6.7 and 6.8 show the AC analysis waveforms. 3dB bandwidths of 2.2GHz and 440MHz are observed for voltage and current transfers, respectively. The gain variability feature of the proposed DC-EXCCII is verified by performing the DC and transient analyses again for different values of DCW, that is, 1000, 1100, 1110 and 1111.

Figures 6.9 and 6.10 depict the gain variability feature of DC-EXCCII through the waveforms obtained by DC and transient analyses, respectively.

Current gain's simulated values for the four cases listed in Table 6.1, are 0.99, 1.98, 2.97 and 3.96, respectively.

6.4 PRACTICABILITY ASPECT OF PROPOSED DC-EXCCII

To verify the applicability of the proposed DC-EXCCII, it is utilized for designing a first order voltage mode (VM) gain controllable APF (GCAPF) from first order VMAPF [31]. The circuit of the GCAPF is shown in Figure 6.11. The DC-EXCCII configuration utilized for realizing the GCAPF, consists of two DCWCs, one for Z_{1p} stage and one for Z_{2n} stage.

The transfer function for the GCAPF is given in Equation 6.2.

$$\frac{V_{out}}{V_{in}} = \left(\frac{R_2}{R_1}\right)\left(\frac{\alpha_{z1p}sR_1C_1 - \alpha_{z2n}}{sR_2C_2 + 1}\right) \tag{6.2}$$

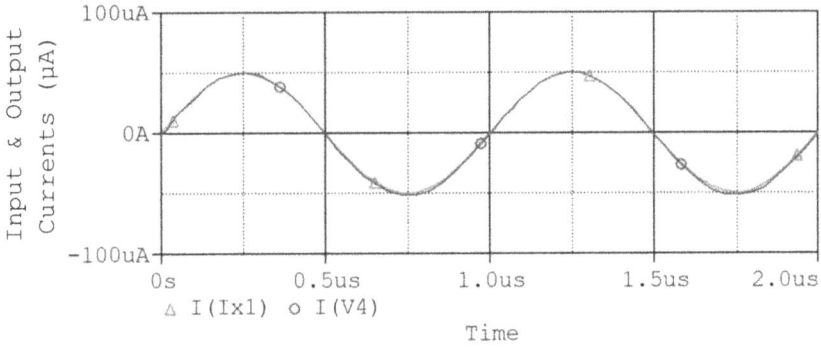

(a)

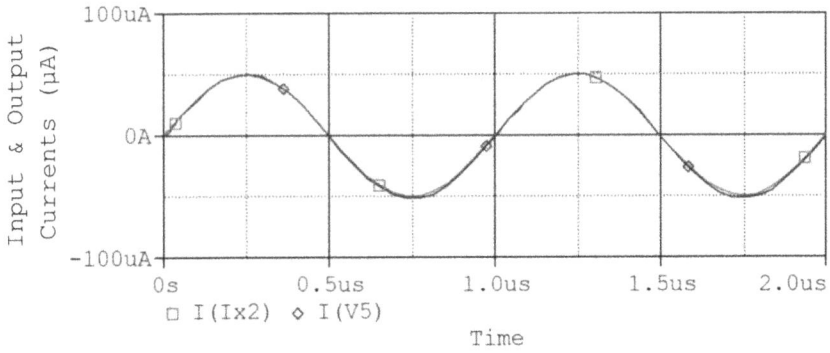

(b)

Figure 6.6 DC-EXCCII time domain current waveforms for unity gain a) X_1 to Z_1 and b) X_2 to Z_2.

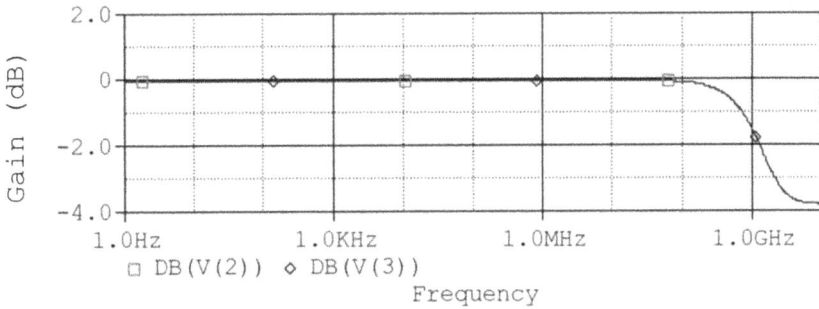

Figure 6.7 DC-EXCCII's frequency response for voltage transfers for unity gain.

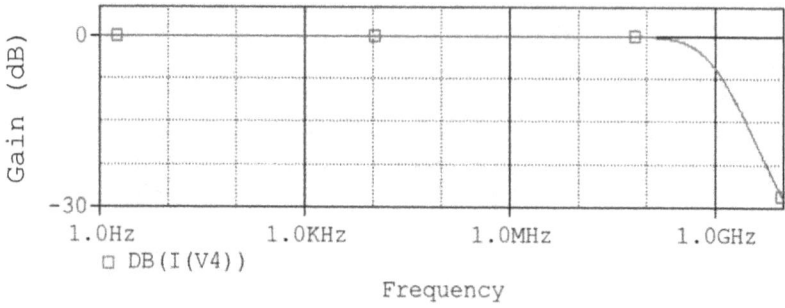

(a)

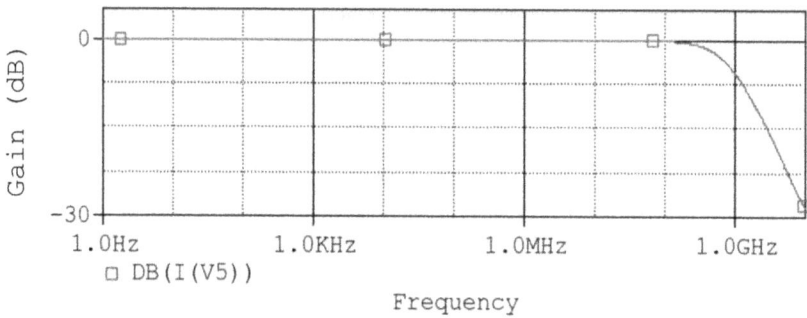

(b)

Figure 6.8 DC-EXCCII's frequency response for current transfers for unity gain a) X_1 to Z_1 and b) X_2 to Z_2.

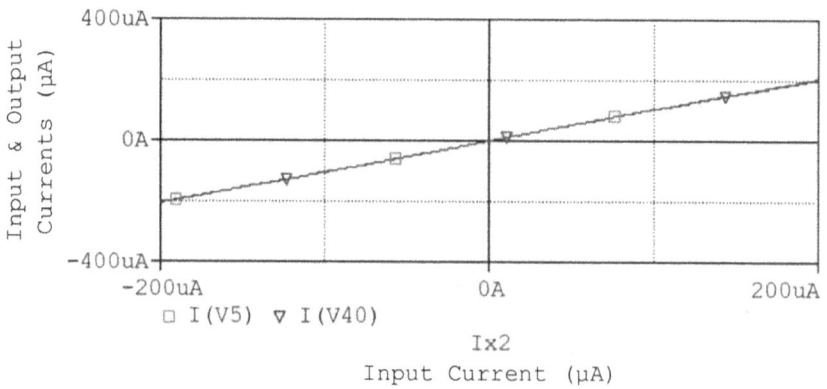

(a)

Figure 6.9 DC-EXCCII's DC analysis for varying DCWs a) 1000

(Continued)

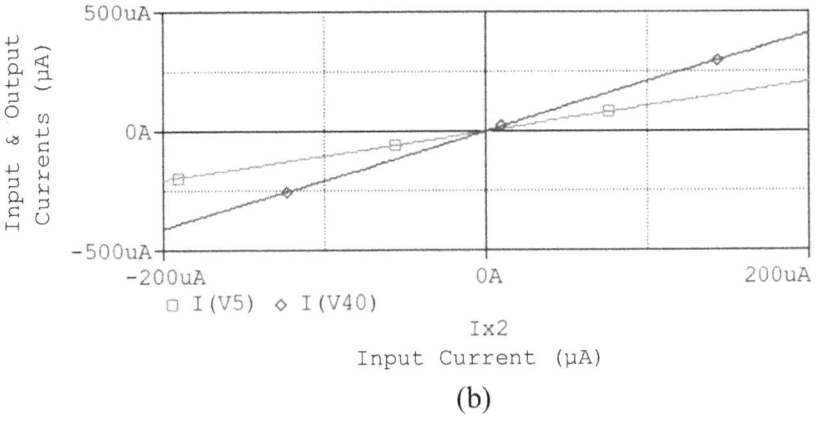

(b)

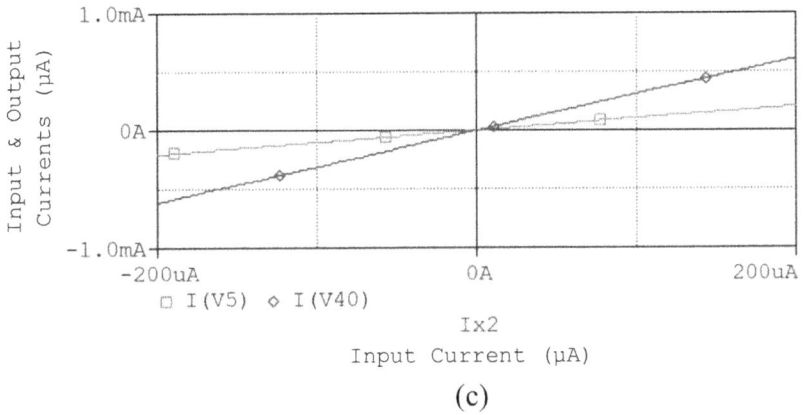

(c)

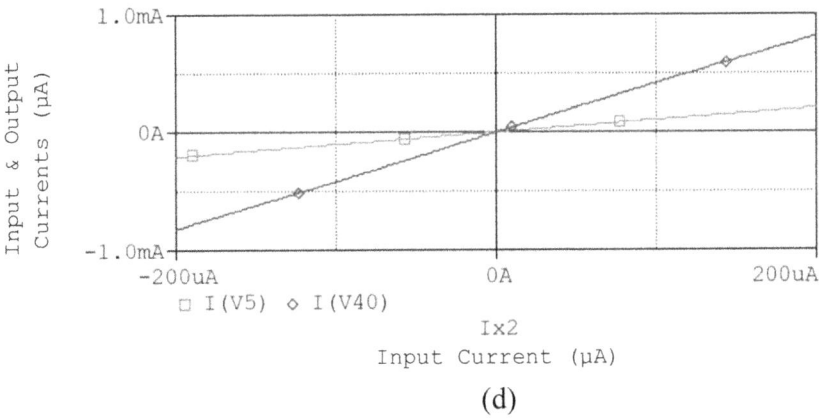

(d)

Figure 6.9 (Continued) DC-EXCCII's DC analysis for varying DCWs b) 1100, c) 1110 and d) 1111.

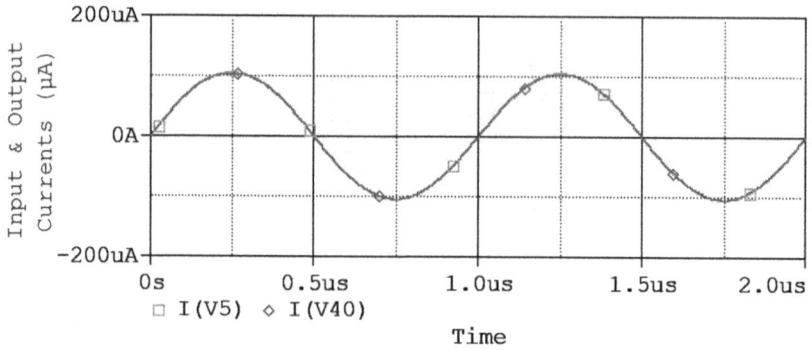

(a)

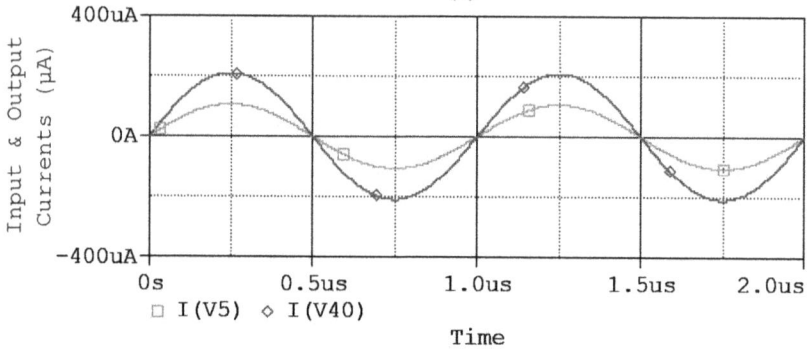

(b)

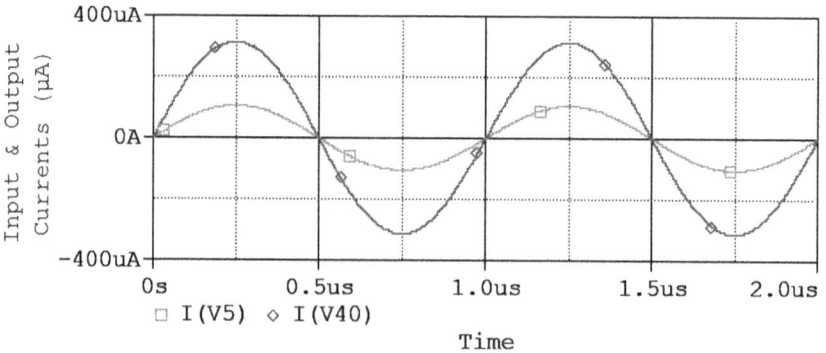

(c)

Figure 6.10 DC-EXCCII's transient analysis for varying DCWs a) 1000, b) 1100, c) 1110 and

(*Continued*)

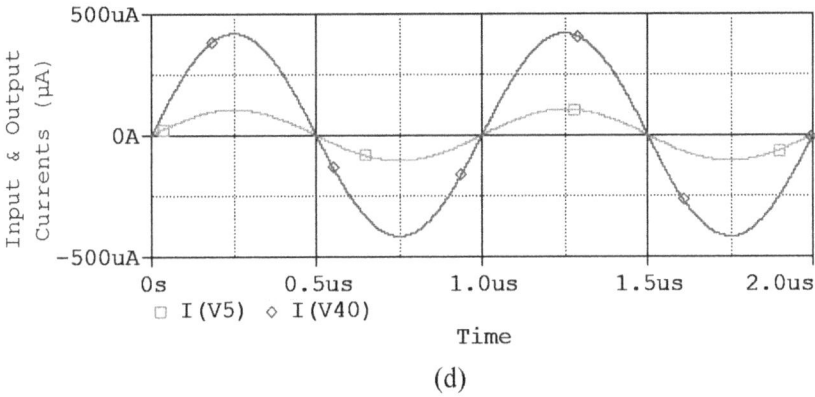

Figure 6.10 (Continued) DC-EXCCII's transient analysis for varying DCWs d) 1111.

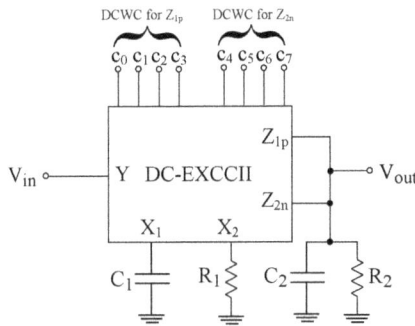

Figure 6.11 DC-EXCCII based GCAPF.

Here, α_{Z1p} and α_{Z2n} are the current transfer gains from port X_1 to Z_{1p} and port X_2 to Z_{2n}, respectively. Using the matched passive components, that is, $C_1=C_2=C$ and $R_1=R_2=R$, Equation 6.2 is updated as expressed below:

$$\frac{V_{out}}{V_{in}} = \frac{\alpha_{Z1p}sRC - \alpha_{Z2n}}{sRC+1} \tag{6.3}$$

Equation 6.3 clearly indicates that the variable AP gain can be achieved by varying α_{Z1p} and α_{Z2n}. This can be done by appropriate selection of the DCWs. Table 6.3 summarizes the realized AP gains for different DCWs setting.

Table 6.3. AP gain variation with varying control words.

S. No.	DCWs Values		GCAPF Gain	Gains for Current Transfer	
	DCW_1 $C_0C_1C_2C_3$	DCW_2 $C_4C_5C_6C_7$		α_{Z1p}	α_{Z2n}
1	1000	1000	1	1	1
2	1100	1100	2	2	2
3	1110	1110	3	3	3
4	1111	1111	4	4	4

Phase angle and pole frequency expressions as observed from Equation 6.3 are given below.

$$\phi = 180° - 2\tan^{-1}(\omega RC) \tag{6.4}$$

$$\omega_0 = \frac{1}{RC} \tag{6.5}$$

Performance verification of GCAPF is done by simulating the circuit on PSPICE at ±1 V supply voltage. In order to validate performance of the proposed idea, the proposed GCAPF has been tested successfully at 3.18MHz operating frequency by choosing R and C values as 5kΩ and 10pF, respectively. The joint phase and gain response for unity AP gain is depicted in Figure 6.12. Gain variability of the AP output is evident from the time domain waveforms shown in Figure 6.13 for different DCWs setting. A noteworthy observation from Figure 6.13 is the unchanged frequency of the output signal, although the gain variation is clearly evident. Simulations indicate power consumption of 0.85mW.

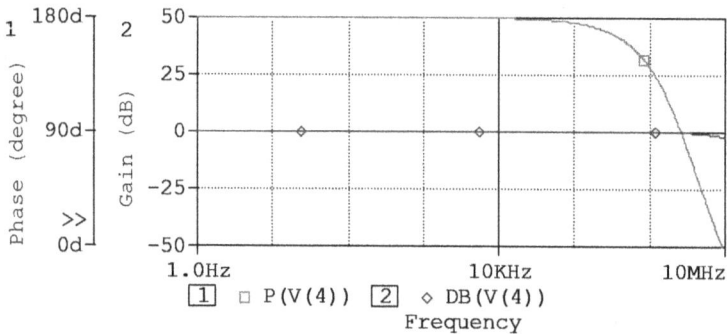

Figure 6.12 Joint phase and gain plots for unity AP gain.

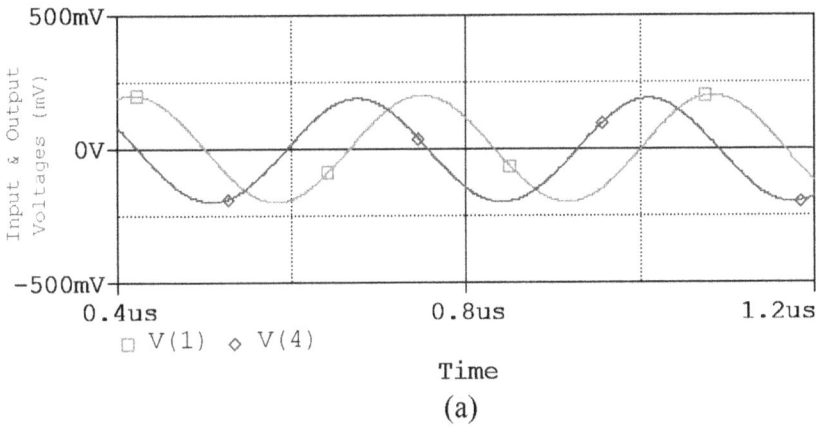

(a)

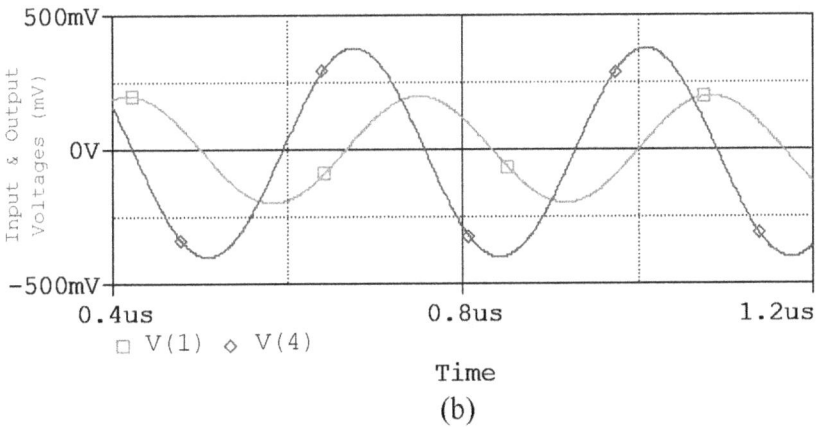

(b)

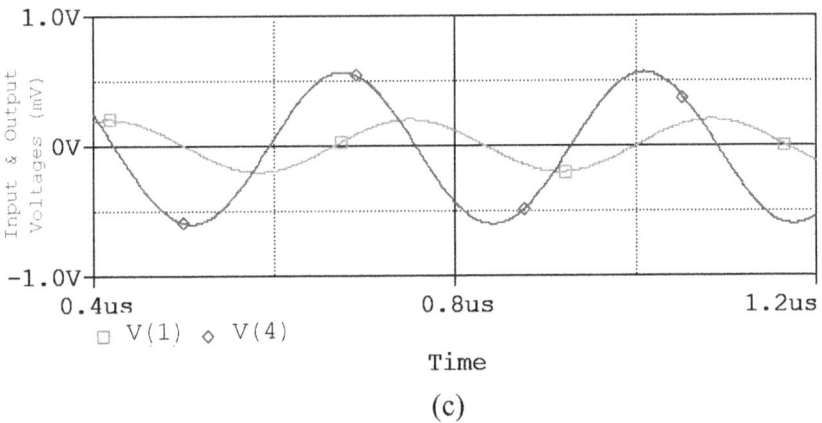

(c)

Figure 6.13 Input and output time domain waveforms for (a) H_{AP} = 1, (b) H_{AP} = 2, (c) H_{AP} = 3

(Continued)

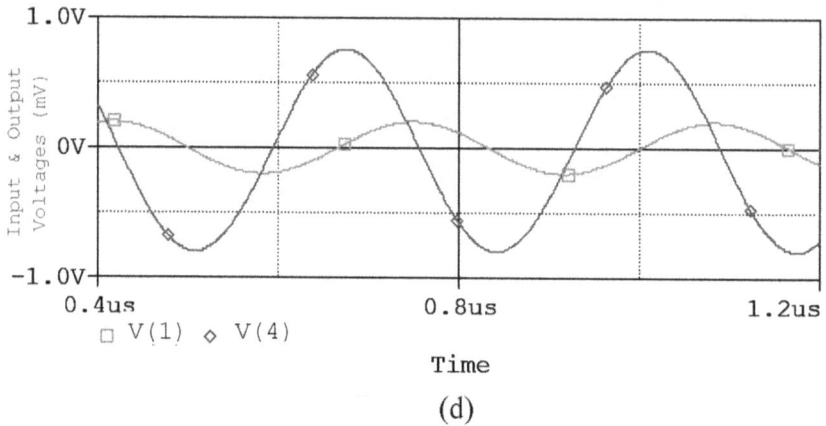

Figure 6.13 (Continued) Input and output time domain waveforms for (d) H_{AP} = 4.

6.5 CONCLUSION

A novel low voltage operated ABB named DC-EXCCII is presented in this chapter. The gain controllability feature is achieved by incorporating a multiple branch DCWC. The DCWC is controlled by a 4-bit DCW which enables or disables the respective DCWC branch(es). The gain variation of the DC-EXCCII lies in the range of 1 to 4. Thereafter, a gain controllable APF is also designed using DC-EXCCII to verify its applicability. The designed APF has high input impedance, low operating voltage, low power dissipation, all grounded passive components and fairly high operating bandwidth. The presented ABB and its APF application are apt choices for biomedical signal processing applications due to its low power requirements. The verification of DC-EXCCII and the designed APF is done through PSPICE simulations conducted at 180nm CMOS technology.

REFERENCES

[1] B. Wilson, "Recent developments in current mode circuits," *IEE Proceedings Circuits, Devices and Systems*, vol. 137, pp. 63–67, 1990.
[2] C. Toumazou, F. J. Lidgey, and D. G. Haigh, *Analogue IC design: The current-mode approach*, Peter Peregrinus Limited, London, 1990.
[3] B. Chaturvedi, A. Kumar, and J. Mohan, "Low voltage operated current-mode first-order universal filter and sinusoidal oscillator suitable for signal processing applications", *AEU International Journal of Electronics and Communications*, vol. 99, pp. 110–118, 2019.
[4] B. Chaturvedi, J. Mohan, A. Kumar, and K. Pal, "Current-mode first order universal filter and it's voltage-mode transformation", *Journal of Circuits, Systems and Computers*, vol. 29, p. 2050149, 2020.

[5] K. C. Smith, and A. S. Sedra, "The current conveyor-A new circuit building block", *Proceedings of the IEEE*, vol. 56, pp. 1368–1369, 1968.

[6] A. S. Sedra, and K. C. Smith, "A second-generation current conveyor and its applications",*IEEE Transactions on Circuit Theory*, vol. 17, pp. 132–134, 1970.

[7] W. Chiu, S. I. Liu, H. W. Tsao, and J. J. Chen, "CMOS differential difference current conveyor and their applications", *IEE Proceedings-Circuits, Devices Systems*, vol. 143, pp. 91–96, 1996.

[8] H. O. Elwan, and A. M. Soliman, "Novel CMOS differential voltage current conveyor and its applications", *IEE Proceedings-Circuits, Devices Systems*, vol. 144, pp. 195–200, 1997.

[9] A. A. El-Adawy, A. M. Soliman, and H. O. Elwan, "A novel fully differential current conveyor and applications for analog VLSI", *IEEE Trans. Circuits and Systems-II: Analog and Digital Signal Processing*, vol. 47, pp. 306–313, 2000.

[10] A. Zeki, and A. Toker, "The dual-X current conveyor (DXCCII): A new active device for tunable continuous-time filters", *International Journal of Electronics*, vol. 89, pp. 913923, 2002.

[11] J. Jitender, J. Mohan, and B. Chaturvedi, "All-pass frequency selective structures: Application for analog domain", *Journal of Circuits, Systems and Computers*, vol. 30 (8), 2150150, 21 Pages, 2021.

[12] B. Chaturvedi, J. Mohan, andA. Kumar, "Resistorless realization of first order current mode universal filter", *Radio Science*, vol. 55, 10 Pages, 2020.

[13] P. Beg, "Tunable first-order resistorless all-pass filter with low-output impedance", *The Scientific World Journal*, vol. 2014, pp. 219453, 2014.

[14] S. Maheshwari, "High performance voltage-mode tunable all-pass section", *Journal of Circuits, Systems, and Computers*, vol. 24, p. 1550080, 2015.

[15] B. Chaturvedi, and A. Kumar, "DXCCTA: A new active element", *IEEE International Conference on Power Electronics, Intelligent Control and Energy Systems (ICPEICES)*, 2016, pp. 1–6.

[16] B. Chaturvedi, and A. Kumar, "CMOS CIDITA and its application", *IEEE International Conference on Power Electronics, Intelligent Control and Energy Systems (ICPEICES)*, 2016, pp. 1–5.

[17] S. A. Mahmoud, and E. A. Soliman, "Digitally programmable second generation current conveyor-based FPAA". *International Journal of Circuit Theory and Applications*, vol. 41, pp. 1074–1084. 2012.

[18] I. A. Khan, M. I. Masud, and S.A. Moiz, "Reconfigurable fully differential first order all pass filter using digitally controlled CMOS DVCC", *Proceedings of the 8th IEEE GCC Conference and Exhibition*, Muscat, Oman, pp. 1–5, 2015.

[19] D. Singh, and N. Afzal, "Digitally programmable high-Q voltage-mode universal filter" *Radioengineering*, vol. 22, pp. 995–1006, 2013.

[20] B. Chaturvedi, J. Mohan, and Jitender, "First order current mode fully cascadable all pass frequency selective structure, it's higher order extension and tunable transformation possibilities", *Journal of Circuits, Systems and Computers*, vol. 31, pp. 2250030, 2022.

[21] J. Jitender, J. Mohan, and B. Chaturvedi, "A novel voltage-mode configuration for first order all-pass filter with one active element and all grounded passive components", *6th International Conference on Signal Processing and Communication (ICSC)*, Noida, pp. 235–239, 2020.

[22] S. Maheshwari, "Some analog filters of reduced complexity with shelving and multifunctional characteristics", *Journal of Circuits, Systems and Computers*, vol. 27, pp.1850150, 2018.

[23] S. Maheshwari, "Tuning approach for first-order filters and new current-mode circuit example", *IET Circuits, Devices and Systems*, vol. 12, pp. 478–485, 2018.

[24] J. Jitender, J. Mohan, and B. Chaturvedi, "CMOS realizable and highly cascadable structures of first-order all-pass filters", Walailak *Journal of Science and Technology*, vol.18 (14), 21451, 19 pages, 2021.

[25] J. Mohan, B. Chaturvedi, and A. Kumar, "New CMOS realizable all pass frequency selective structures", *Journal of Circuits, Systems and Computers*, vol. 30 (15), 2150268, 16 Pages, 2021.

[26] S. Maheshwari, "Current-mode circuit with high output impedance for phase-shifting applications", *International Journal of Electronics and Information Engineering*, vol. 12, pp. 16–23, 2020.

[27] J. Mohan, B. Chaturvedi, and Jitender, "CMOS compatible first order current mode universal filter structure and its possible tunable variant", *Journal of Circuits, Systems and Computers*, vol. 31, p. 2250242, 2022.

[28] Fatemeh KaramiHorestani, Z. K. Horastani, and N. Björsell, "A band-pass instrumentation amplifier based on a differential voltage current conveyor for biomedical signal recording applications", *Electronics*, vol. 11, p.1087, 2022.

[29] M. Kumngern, F. Khateb, and T. Kulej, "0.5 V current-mode low-pass filter based on voltage second generation current conveyor for bio-sensor applications," *IEEE Access*, vol. 10, pp. 12201–12207, 2022.

[30] T. M. Hassan, and S. A. Mahmoud, "Fully programmable universal filter with independent gain-ω_0-Q control based on new digitally programmable CMOS CCII", *Journal of Circuits, Systems and Computers*, vol. 18, pp. 875–897, 2009.

[31] J. Jitender, J. Mohan, and B. Chaturvedi, "A novel voltage-mode configuration for first order all-pass filter with one active element and all grounded passive components", *6th International Conference on Signal Processing and Communication (ICSC)*, Noida, pp. 235–239, 2020.

Chapter 7

Study of Analog Filters Employing Current-Mode Active Elements Suitable for Biomedical Applications

Priyanka Singh, Vikas Tiwari and
Rajendra Kumar Nagaria
Motilal Nehru National Institute of Technology, Allahabad, India

CONTENTS

ABBREVIATIONS

AP	All pass
BP	Band pass
BR	Band reject
CC	Current conveyor
CM	Current mode
CMOS	Complementary MOSFET
DV-EXCCCII	Differential voltage extra-X current controlled current conveyor
HP	High pass
IC	Integrated circuit
LP	Low pass
MOSFET	Metal oxide field effect transistor
UF	Universal filter
VLSI	Very large scale integration
VM	Voltage mode
Vth	Threshold voltage

DOI: 10.1201/9781003431138-7

7.1 INTRODUCTION

The need for portable devices is increasing and the power dissipation involved in designing these circuits is one of the numerous difficulties an analog designer must overcome. Lowering the supply voltage is an easy way to cut down on power usage, but doing so will have an impact on the system's bandwidth, slew rate and noise. It is important to note that the scaling of technology node aids in lowering both the supply voltage and the metal oxide field effect transistor's (MOSFET) threshold voltage (V_{th}) [1, 2]. While using the body biasing technique, a designer can further adjust the MOSFET's V_{th} to meet design requirements. But doing so will raise the system's leakage current, which is a significant issue at lower supply voltage. Biomedical devices employ filters to pass low frequency signals and these are further passed to an analog to cigital converter. The voltage-mode (VM) approach is the foundation for the traditional analog system design. At greater supply voltages and lower operating frequencies, voltage-mode circuits perform very well, but at lower technology nodes and higher frequencies, their performance suffers. These issues are mostly brought on by their high output impedance, which limits the system's output swing. An alternative remedy for the aforementioned problems is the current-mode (CM) approach, which operates at a lower supply voltage [3]. The CM circuits have many advantages over VM in terms of gain, bandwidth, slew rate, linearity and power consumption among others. In current-mode circuits, the branch currents are the main design parameters rather than nodal voltages. Thus, current-mode (CM) circuits offer greater potential in combating the difficulties which arise due to the reduction in supply voltage. The above-mentioned features of current-mode circuits make them a popular choice of circuit designers to enable them to realize low-voltage and low-power circuits with high speed and wider bandwidth.

Nowadays, in modern microelectronics and very large scale integration (VLSI) design, current conveyors (CC) are the most noticeable high performance current-mode active elements available in the literature [4]. The current conveyors comprise both voltage and current sub-blocks, and they are found to be very suitable in the design of high speed and high frequency CM as well as VM circuits. Current conveyors provide an attractive alternative to op-amp in both VM and CM applications. It is well known that commonly used integrated circuit (IC) technologies are bipolar and complementary-MOSFET (CMOS). The current conveyors have been implemented in both bipolar and CMOS technologies. Thus, the feasibility of current conveyors in modern IC technologies has made them more popular in realizing signal processing functions. Modifications to the basic conveyors has resulted in the development of a variety of new conveyors. A variety of applications based on current conveyors and their variants have been reported in the literature.

With the improvement in the CM design approach, several CM active building blocks are introduced in the literature [4–34]. Some of the mostly used current-mode active blocks are CCII [4], DVCC [5, 6], CCII-TA [7], DX-MOCCII [10], MOCCII [11], ICCII [13], CDTA [14], EX-CCCII [16], VDCC [18], CCCII [21, 22], CCDDCC [25], CCCCTA [27], OFCC [28, 29], DV-EXCCCII [34] and many more. These current-mode active elements are used to design many analog signal processing modules to enhance the performance of the circuit.

7.2 CURRENT-MODE ANALOG FILTERS

Analog filter design is one of the important research subjects in the CM approach. Filters are essential building blocks in several applications, such as communication systems, analog signal processing, and instrumentation systems, among others [5–34]. A filter is basically a device designed to isolate, suppress or pass a group of signals from unwanted signals. Various first- and second-order filters composed of different CM elements are reported in the literature.

The circuit design using electronically tunable current-mode block is preferred. The parameters of the circuit depend on the value of passive components used in the circuit. These passive elements are a function of aging, temperature, humidity, process tolerance and so forth. As a result, the circuit's performance deviates from the nominal design. Therefore, there is increasing interest in designing electronically tunable circuits to compensate for deviation caused by process tolerance, parasitic, temperature drift, and component aging. Many circuits reported in the literature do have electronic tuning capability. A brief study is presented of analog filters employing various current-mode building blocks.

7.2.1 First-Order Filters Based on Current-Mode Approach

In literature, various first-order filters are discussed based on CM elements. The VM high input impedance first-order universal filters (UF) composed of DVCC are proposed in [5, 6]. The low pass (LP), high pass (HP) and all-pass (AP) signals can be achieved simultaneously using the same topology. The circuit given in [5] employs one DVCC, and three passive elements whereas, the circuit given in [6] uses two DVCCs, and two passive elements. A first-order multi-function filter based on CCII-TA is reported in [7]. Only one active element and four passive elements are used in the suggested circuit. The electronic tuning of the suggested filter is achieved by adjusting the bias current. This circuit is suitable for integration. It uses one grounded capacitor and three resistors, and can realize LP, HP and AP filters.

A novel first-order VM filter composed of minimum components is reported in [8]. The suggested structure requires one DVCC, and two passive elements to realize the filter response. This filter can provide simultaneously first-order LP, HP and AP filters. The CCII based novel filter employing five passive elements is discussed in [9]. The circuit's architecture can also be alternatively designed with CCCII. This variant of the circuit allows for electronic tuning of the cutoff frequency while also reducing component count by using only one capacitor and two resistors rather than five passive elements. The circuit enjoys low sensitivity figures.

A CM universal filter based on ICCIIs is discussed in [13]. The suggested circuit is resistor-less and employs two ICCII and a capacitor to realize all the filter responses. This circuit realizes inverting and non-inverting LP, HP, and AP filters simultaneously without passive element matching condition. This circuit is electronically tunable because a transistor is working in the linear region, which can be considered as a variable resistor to control the response of the filter. A new CM first-order AP based on two CDTA and a single capacitor is reported in [14]. It can provide inverting and non-inverting AP without matching constraints. This circuit is resistor-less and cascadable.

A novel CM universal filter based on DO-CCIIs, and two passive components is reported in [15]. This circuit is cascadable without additional buffer requirements. It can provide LP and AP simultaneously, and HP by combining the outputs of LP and AP without any matching constraints. The electronic tuning of the circuit can be achieved by using DO-CCCIIs instead of DO-CCIIs. The resultant circuit is represented in Figure 7.1.

An electronically tunable filter [16] is represented in Figure 7.2. This filter is based on one EX-CCCII and a capacitor. It requires a single input current signal and provides LP, HP and AP filters simultaneously at different output terminals. Due to grounded passive element the circuit is appropriate for integration. This filter is cascadable and has electronic tuning capability.

7.2.2 Second-Order Filters Based on Current-Mode Approach

Second-order active filters are the most widely used filters and are used as fundamental elements for higher-order filters. A large volume of work

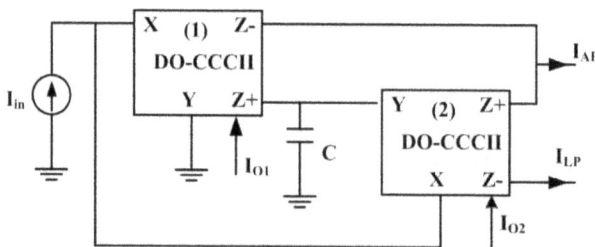

Figure 7.1 The current-mode filter using DO-CCCII [15]. Two DO-CCCIIs are used to obtain a universal filter.

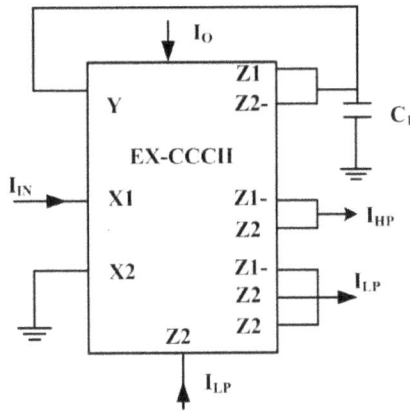

Figure 7.2 The CM filter based on EX-CCCII [16]. Single EX-CCCII used to obtain universal filter.

on the subject is available in the literature. A biquadratic filter employing current-conveyor is proposed in [17]. It can provide LP, HP, AP, BP (band-pass), and BR (band-reject) filters. It employs seven CCs and two capacitors and four resistors. It is appropriate for integration. To implement the filter, more components are employed which increases the area. Two VM and two CM universal biquadratic filters are reported in [18]. These are composed of one VDCC, and four passive elements. The LP, HP, AP, BP and BR filters are realized from the same circuit topology. Furthermore, the reported filters do not need any double/inverted input signals to implement the circuit. Also, the sensitivities are found to be low.

A novel CM biquadratic filter based on DVCC is discussed in [19]. This filter is composed of three DVCCs, two capacitors and three resistors. The proposed filter can be configured in two ways. The first topology provides BP, HP and BR outputs simultaneously, whereas the second topology provides both inverted and non-inverted type LP, HP, BP, AP and BR outputs by appropriate selection of inputs. The response of this circuit can be controlled independently by tuning the grounded passive components. All of the filter outputs can be realized without any matching constraints. Another electronically tunable CM universal biquadratic filter based on two DVCCs is proposed in [20]. This can realize LP, BP and notch outputs at a high output impedance terminal simultaneously by using two equal input signals. In addition, by combining the proper output signals, it can also provide HP and AP. The limitation of the circuit is that more active and passive elements are needed to obtain the filter responses and also component matching is needed. In addition, a floating resistor is used, which is not suitable for integration.

A new CM biquadratic universal filter circuit employing five CCII+s, three resistors and three capacitors [21] is depicted in Figure 7.3. This configuration

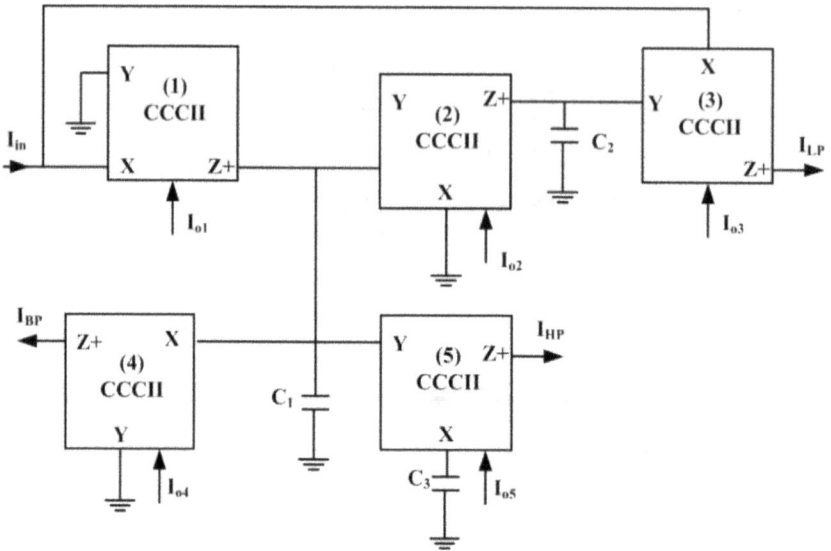

Figure 7.3 The block diagram of CM filter reported in [21]. Five CCCII used for resistorless filter.

can provide HP, BP and LP filter responses at the same time. It can also provide AP and notch filter responses by combining the proper output signals. The electronically tunable version of the circuit can be obtained by replacing CCII+s with plus type CCCII and removing all three resistors. However, it needs matching constraints for notch and AP filter.

Two electronically tunable CM second-order universal filters [22] depicted in Figure 7.4 can realize LP, BP and HP responses. These circuits can also provide notch and AP by combining the appropriate outputs. The first circuit employs two single output CCCIIs and two dual output CCCIIs, whereas the second circuit uses five single output CCCIIs. These circuits are resistor-less and use only grounded capacitors.

A novel current-controlled CM biquadratic filter is represented in Figure 7.5. The reported circuit is composed of two CCCIIs, one MO-CCCA and two capacitors [23]. This configuration can provide LP, HP, AP, BP and BR responses. Furthermore, the filter response has an independent electronic tuning feature with the bias current of CCCIIs. Furthermore, by altering the value of bias currents of MO-CCCA, a high value of quality factor of the reported filter may easily be obtained. The sensitivities of parameters are found to be low in magnitude.

A current-controlled CM biquadratic UF composed of two CCCCTAs and two capacitors [24] is shown in Figure 7.6. This filter provides LP, HP, BP, AP and BR responses. The circuit response can be adjusted with the bias current without changing the value of pole frequency. The current controlled UF

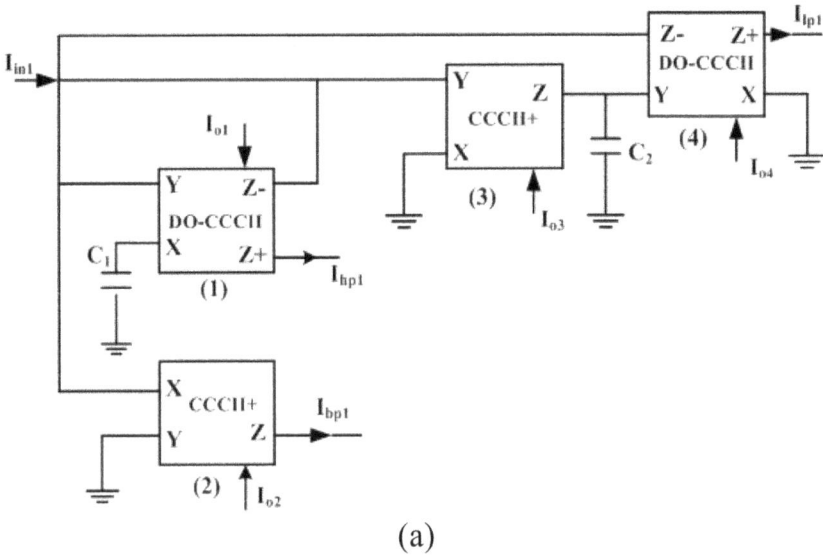

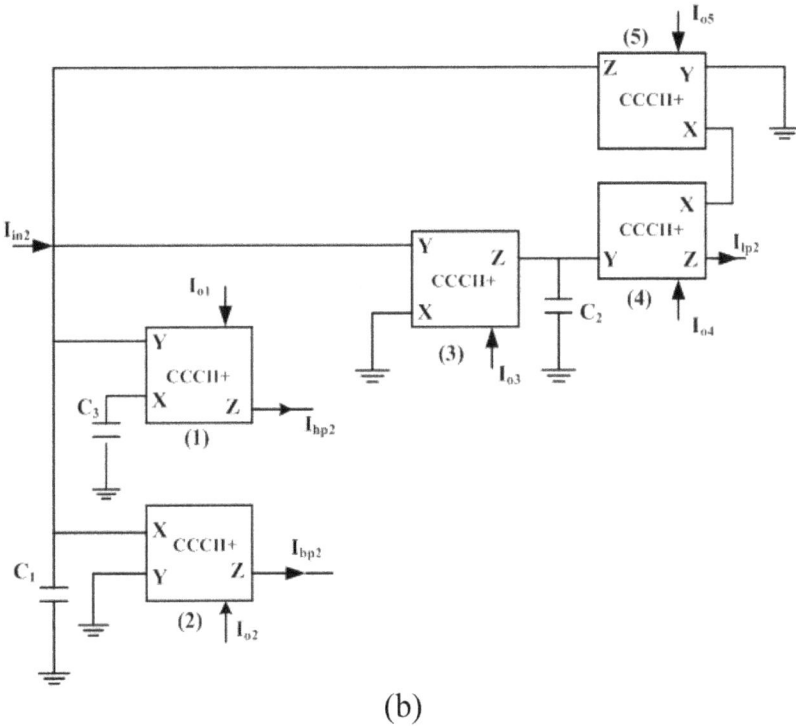

Figure 7.4 The biquadratic universal filter of [22]. (a) Topology 1 (b) Topology 2. An electronically tunable filter is obtained using CCCII.

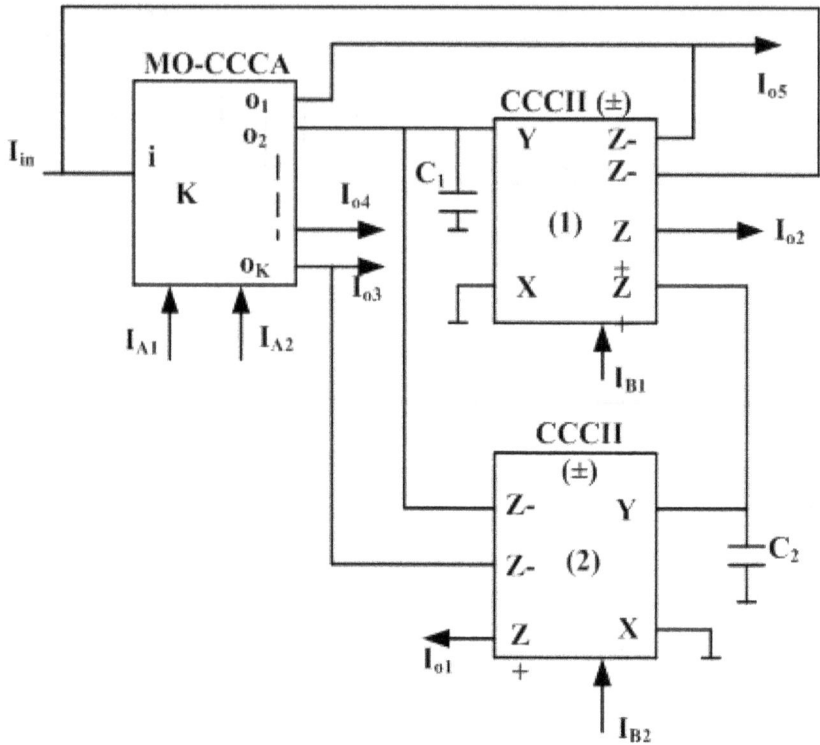

Figure 7.5 The block diagram of a filter based on CCCII and MO-CCCA [23]. A current controlled filter is obtained using two CCCIIs and one MO-CCCA.

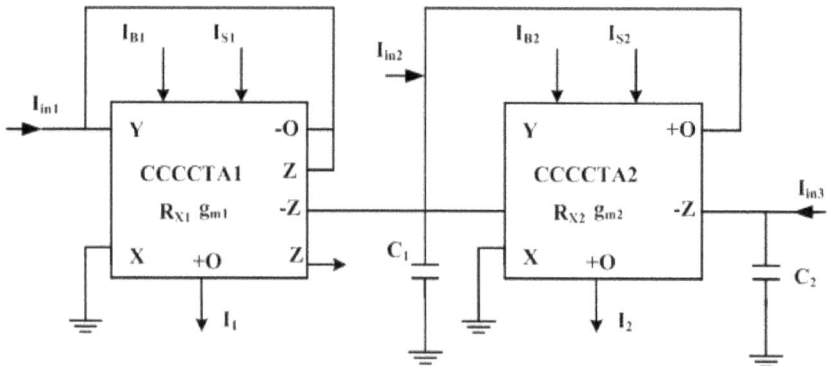

Figure 7.6 The current controlled filter employing CCCCTA [24]. A current-controlled CM filter composed of two CCCCTAs and two capacitors is used to obtain biquadratic LP, HP, AP, BP, and BR filters.

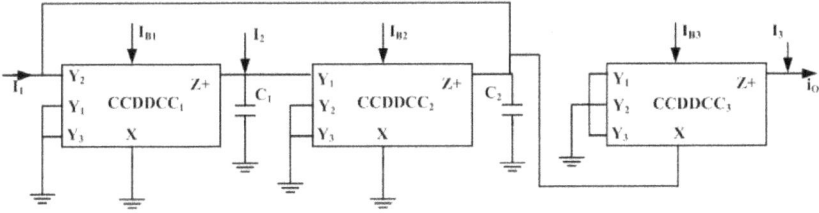

Figure 7.7 The universal biquadratic filter based on CCDDCC [25]. Three CCDDCCs and two capacitors are used to obtain biquadratic LP, HP, AP, BP, and BR filters.

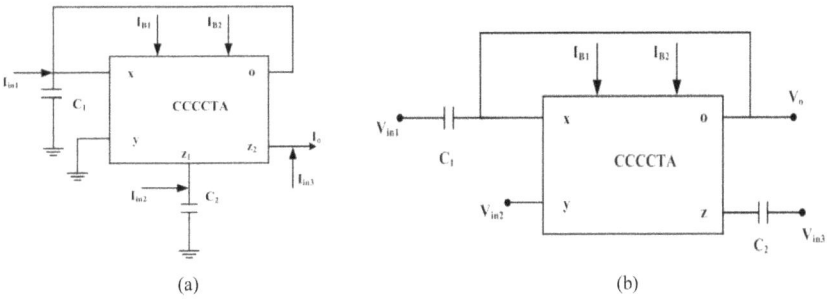

(a)   (b)

Figure 7.8 (a) CM (b) VM filters based on CCCCTA [27]. A single CCCCTA is used to obtain CM and VM filters.

composed of three CCDDCCs and two capacitors is depicted in Figure 7.7 [25]. The filter offers LP, HP, AP, BP and notch filters simultaneously.

A CM and a VM biquadratic filter is proposed in [27] employing a single CCCCTA. The reported current-mode circuit is depicted in Figure 7.8 (a). This circuit can realize all filter responses depending on the digital selection, without altering circuit structure. The proposed voltage-mode biquadratic circuit employing a single CCCCTA is shown in Figure 7.8 (b). It requires matching conditions to implement the circuit. The comparative study of various reported biquadratic universal filter is shown in Table 7.1.

7.3 SECOND-ORDER UNIVERSAL FILTER BASED ON DV-EXCCCII

An electronically tunable second-order CM universal filter designed with a single DV-EXCCCII is proposed in [34]. This CM biquadratic filter provides LP, HP, AP, BP and BR responses. This filter is implemented using one resistor and two capacitors and is suitable for cascading.

Table 7.1 Comparative study of biquadratic filters based on CM active elements

Reference	ABB type	No. of ABBs	Number of resistors		Number of capacitors		Tunability	Technology (μm)	Power supplies (V)	Matching required
			Floating	Grounded	Floating	Grounded				
Chen [19]	DVCC	3	0	3	0	2	Yes	0.18	± 0.9	No
Abaci and Yuce [20]	DVCC	2	1	2	0	2	Yes	0.13	± 0.75	Yes
Yucel and Yuce [21]	CCCII	5	0	0	0	3	Yes	0.13	± 0.75	Yes
Yuce and Minaei [22]	CCCII	5	0	0	0	3	Yes	BJT	± 2.5	No
Nand and Pandey [28]	OFCC	3	0	3	0	2	Yes	0.5	± 1.5	No
Pandey et al. [29]	OFCC	3	0	2	0	2	Yes	0.5	± 1.5	No
Horng [30]	MOCCII	3	0	3	0	2	No	0.35	± 1.65	No
Horng [31]	MOCCII	3	2	3	0	2	No	0.18	± 1.25	No
Hassen et al. [32]	ICCII	3	0	4	0	2	No	0.18	± 0.8	No
Kacar et al. [33]	FDCCII	1	0	2	0	2	No	0.35	± 1.3	No

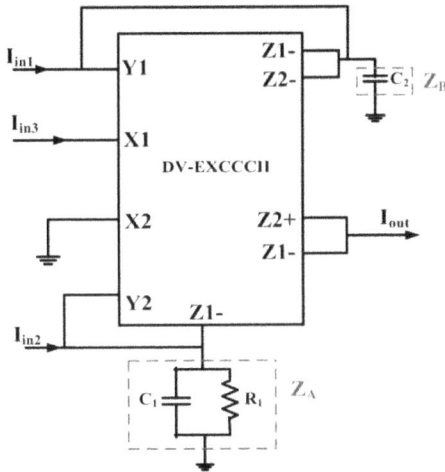

Figure 7.9 The DV-EXCCCII based universal filter [34]. A second-order universal filter is obtained using a single DV-EXCCCII.

7.3.1 Circuit Description

Figure 7.9 displays the block diagram of a biquadratic filter with a single DV-EXCCCII reported in [34]. The output current is calculated as,

$$
I_{out} = \frac{I_{in1}\left(1 + R_1C_1s\right) - I_{in2}R_1C_2s + I_{in3}\left[R_1R_{X2}C_1C_2s^2 + R_{X2}C_2s + 2R_1C_1s - R_1C_2s + 2\right]}{\left(R_1C_1s + 1\right)\left(R_{X2}C_2s + 1\right)}
$$

(7.1)

Equation 7.1 can realize all filters using different input combinations. Table 7.2 shows the input combinations used for each filter taking $C_1 = C_2$, $R_{X2} = R_1$.

Table 7.2 Input combinations for realization of second-order universal filter

Second order filter response	Input combination		
	I_{in1}	I_{in2}	I_{in3}
Low Pass	1	1	0
High Pass	−2	0	1
All Pass	1	−3	−1
Band Pass	0	1	0
Band Reject	−1	1	1

The filter parameters are determined as,

$$\text{Pole frequency} = \frac{1}{2\pi\sqrt{R_1 R_{X2} C_1 C_2}} \tag{7.2}$$

$$\text{Bandwidth} = \frac{1}{R_1 C_1} + \frac{1}{R_{X2} C_2} \tag{7.3}$$

$$\text{Quality factor} = \frac{\sqrt{R_1 R_{X2} C_1 C_2}}{R_1 C_1 + R_{X2} C_2} \tag{7.4}$$

7.3.2 Simulation Result

The electronically tunable filter represented in Figure 7.9 is simulated using 0.18 μm technology at ±0.9 V supply. Figures 7.10 and 7.11 show the frequency response of the filter shown in [34] for different capacitor values. The Monte Carlo histogram for the DV-EXCCCII based filter is shown in Figure 7.12. The tunability characteristic of the filter is represented in Figure 7.13. The power dissipation of the circuit is observed as 2.2 mW.

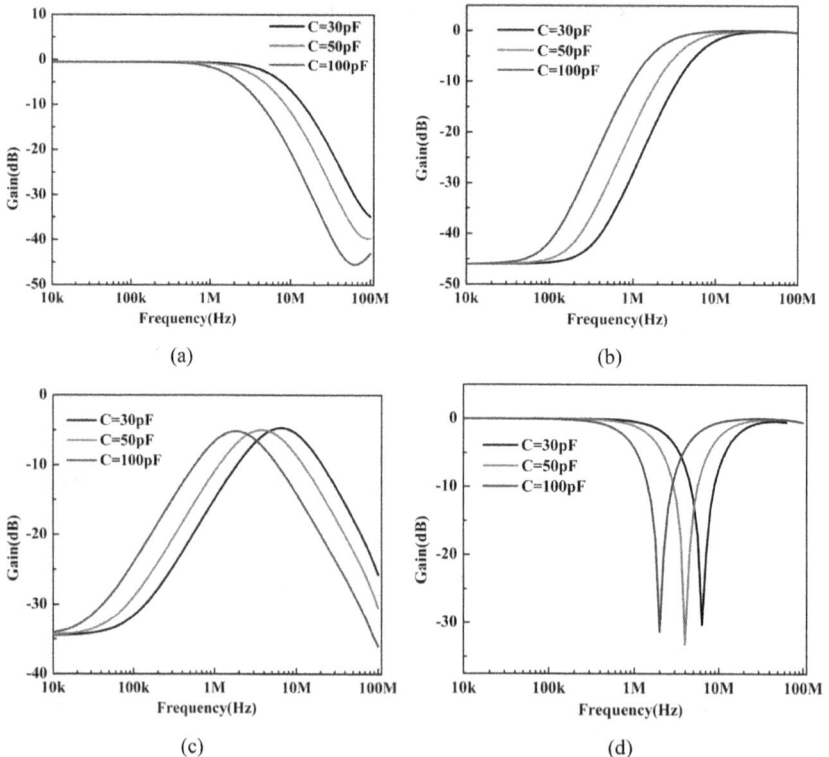

Figure 7.10 Magnitude response for (a) LP (b) HP (c) BP (d) BR filters.

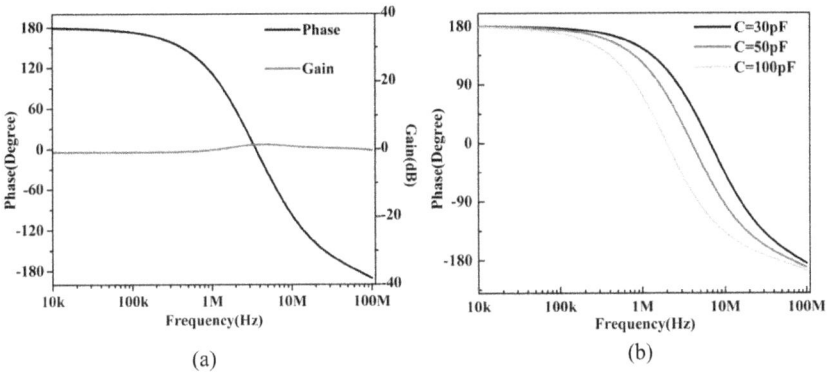

Figure 7.11 (a) Frequency response (b) Phase variation for various capacitors for AP filter.

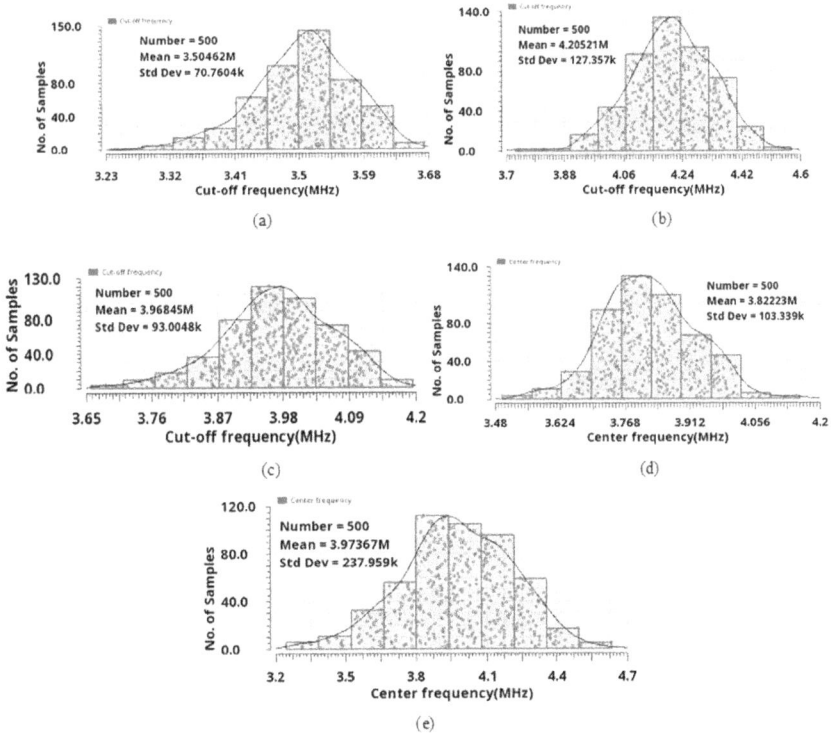

Figure 7.12 Monte-Carlo histograms for (a) LP (b) HP (c) AP (d) BP (e) BR filters.

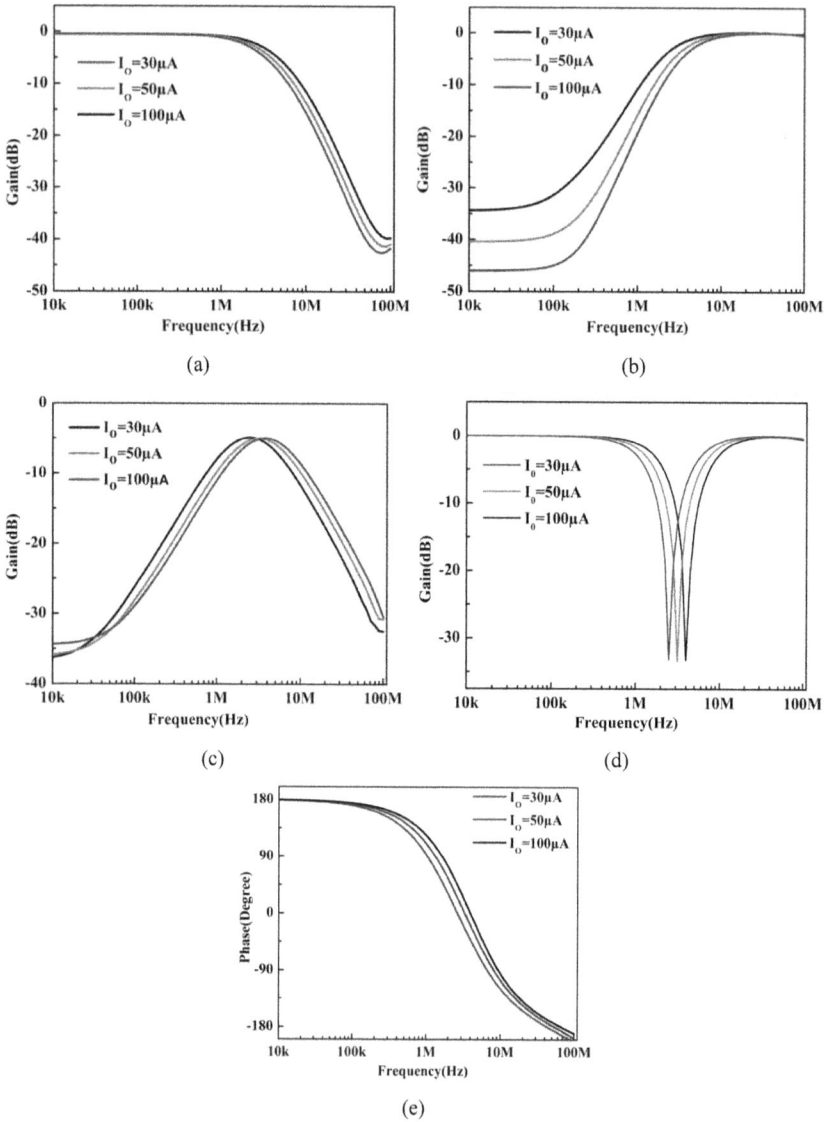

Figure 7.13 Frequency response at different bias currents for (a) LP (b) HP (c) BP (d) BR (e) AP filters.

Table 7.3 represents the pole frequency for different capacitor values and Table 7.4 shows the pole frequency for several bias currents. Table 7.5 shows the values of pole frequency of AP for different corners, voltages and temperatures. Noise immunity of the circuit is investigated next. Values of

Table 7.3 Pole frequency for various capacitors

C (pF)	Pole frequency (MHz)				
	LP	HP	AP	BP	BR
C = 30	6	7	6.4	6.3	6.8
C = 50	3.5	4.2	3.95	3.8	4
C = 100	1.6	2.2	2	1.9	2

Table 7.4 Pole frequency for various bias currents

I_o (μA)	Pole frequency (MHz)				
	LP	HP	AP	BP	BR
I_o = 30	2.2	2.5	2.5	2.5	2.5
I_o = 50	2.4	2.9	3.1	2.9	3.1
I_o = 100	3.5	4.2	3.95	3.8	4

Table 7.5 Pole frequency of AP for different corners, voltages and temperatures

Variation	Different values	Pole frequency (MHz)
Process	Typical	3.95
	FF	4.23
	FNSP	3.89
	SNFP	3.91
	SS	3.71
Voltage	$V_{DD} = -V_{ss} = 0.85$	3.49
	$V_{DD} = -V_{ss} = 0.9$	3.95
	$V_{DD} = -V_{ss} = 0.95$	4.35
Temperature	$-50°C$	4.46
	$0°C$	4.12
	$50°C$	3.85
	$100°C$	3.79
	$150°C$	3.23

Table 7.6 Noise at various corners for different frequencies at 100μA bias current

Frequency	Input noise (I_N) (A/√Hz) Output noise (O_N) (V/√Hz)	Typical	FF	Different process corners FNSP	SNFP	SS
1 Hz	I_N	1.23×10^{-6}	8.50×10^{-7}	8.69×10^{-7}	1.39×10^{-6}	1.48×10^{-6}
	O_N	1.47×10^{-5}	1.63×10^{-5}	1.52×10^{-5}	1.49×10^{-5}	1.36×10^{-5}
1 KHz	I_N	4.26×10^{-8}	3.9×10^{-8}	3.3×10^{-8}	5.8×10^{-8}	5.5×10^{-8}
	O_N	6.32×10^{-7}	7.20×10^{-7}	6.83×10^{-7}	6.25×10^{-7}	5.16×10^{-7}
100 KHz	I_N	2.87×10^{-9}	2.95×10^{-9}	2.49×10^{-9}	2.86×10^{-9}	2.22×10^{-9}
	O_N	7.85×10^{-8}	8.26×10^{-8}	7.24×10^{-8}	7.07×10^{-8}	6.42×10^{-8}
1 MHz	I_N	1.32×10^{-10}	1.35×10^{-10}	1.81×10^{-10}	1.62×10^{-10}	9.42×10^{-11}
	O_N	2.83×10^{-8}	3.36×10^{-8}	2.39×10^{-8}	3.20×10^{-8}	2.16×10^{-8}
100 MHz	I_N	4.41×10^{-10}	3.79×10^{-10}	4.31×10^{-10}	4.71×10^{-10}	4.63×10^{-10}
	O_N	1.25×10^{-8}	1.56×10^{-8}	1.64×10^{-8}	1.75×10^{-8}	1.73×10^{-8}

input and output noise at various corners for different frequencies at 100μA bias current are represented in Table 7.6.

7.4 CONCLUSION

In this chapter, an overview of analog filters using various current-mode active building blocks is presented. A large volume of work on the subject employing current-mode approach is available in the literature. From the above discussion, it is noted that they suffer from several imperfections. Many circuits reported in the literature employ more active and passive elements which increases the complexity and area of the circuits. Many in the reported work do not employ electronically tunable current controlled active elements, and some circuits require matching condition to realize the response of the circuit. Many circuits do not have appropriate output impedance and, therefore, require additional circuits while cascading with other current-mode circuits. A brief comparison of some reported second-order filters is also presented. The simulation results of DV-EXCCCII based biquadratic universal filters are also discussed.

REFERENCES

1. Razavi, B., *Design of analog CMOS integrated circuits*, 1st ed. New Delhi, India: Tata McGraw Hill, 2005.
2. Bahramali, A. and Lopez-Vallejo, M., "A low power RFID based energy harvesting temperature resilient CMOS-only reference voltage", *Integration the VLSI Journal*, vol. 67, pp. 155–161, 2019.
3. Toumazou, C., Lidgey, F. J., and Haigh, D., *Analogue IC design: the current-mode approach*, vol. 2, Presbyterian Publishing Corp, 1990.
4. Sedra, A. S., and Smith, K., "A second-generation current conveyor and its applications", *IEEE Transactions on Circuit Theory*, vol. 17, no. 1, pp. 132–134, 1970.
5. Horng, J. W., "High input impedance first-order allpass, highpass and low-pass filters with grounded capacitor using single DVCC", *Indian Journal of Engineering and Materials Sciences*, vol. 17, pp. 175–178, 2010.
6. Horng, J. W., "DVCCs based high input impedance voltage-mode first-order allpass, highpass and lowpass filters employing grounded capacitor and resistor", *Radioengineering*, vol. 19, no. 4, pp. 653–656, 2010.
7. Pandey, N., Kapur, S., Arora, P., and Malhotra, S., "Novel voltage mode multifunction filter based on current conveyor transconductance amplifier", *International Journal on Control System and Instrumentation*, vol. 2, no. 1, pp. 42–45, 2011.
8. Chen, H. P., Huang, K. W., and Huang, P. M., "DVCC-based first-order filter with grounded capacitor", *International Journal of Information and Electronics Engineering*, vol. 2, no. 1, pp. 50–54, 2012.

9. Shah, N. A., Iqbal, S. Z., and Parveen, B., "Simple first-order multifunction filter", *Indian Journal of Pure and Applied Physics*, vol. 42, pp. 854–856, 2004.

10. Beg, P., Siddiqi, M. A., and Ansari, M. S., "Multi output filter and four phase sinusoidal oscillator using CMOS DX-MOCCII", *International Journal of Electronics*, vol. 98, no. 9, pp. 1185–1198, 2011.

11. Khan, I. A., Beg, P., and Ahmed, M. T., "First order current mode filters and multiphase sinusoidal oscillators using CMOS MOCCIIs", *Arabian Journal for Science and Engineering*, vol. 32, no. 2, pp. 119–126, 2007.

12. Kumar, A., and Paul, S. K., "Current mode first order universal filter and multiphase sinusoidal oscillator", *AEU-International Journal of Electronics and Communications*, vol. 81, pp. 37–49, 2017.

13. Safari, L., Yuce, E., and Minaei, S., "A new ICCII based resistor-less current-mode first-order universal filter with electronic tuning capability", *Microelectronics Journal*, vol. 67, pp. 101–110, 2017.

14. Tangsrirat, W., Pukkalanun, T., and Surakampontorn, W., "Resistorless realization of current-mode first-order allpass filter using current differencing transconductance amplifiers", *Microelectronics Journal*, vol. 41, no. (2–3), pp. 178–183, 2010.

15. Yuce, E., and Minaei, S., "A first-order fully cascadable current-mode universal filter composed of dual output CCIIs and a grounded capacitor", *Journal of Circuits, Systems and Computers*, vol. 25, no. 5, 1650042, 2016.

16. Agrawal, D., and Maheshwari, S., "An active-C current-mode universal first-order filter and oscillator", *Journal of Circuits, Systems and Computers*, vol. 28, no. 13, 1950219, 2019.

17. Senani, R., "New current-mode biquad filter", *International Journal of Electronics*, vol. 73, no. 4, pp. 735–742, 1992.

18. Roy, S., Paul, T. K., Maiti, S., and Pal, R. R., "Voltage differencing current conveyor based voltage-mode and current-mode universal biquad filters with electronic tuning facility", *International Journal of Engineering and Technology Innovation*, vol. 11, no. 2, pp. 146–160, 2021.

19. Chen, H. P., "Tunable versatile current-mode universal filter based on plus-type DVCCs", *AEU-International Journal of Electronics and Communications*, vol. 66, no. 4, pp. 332–339, 2012.

20. Abaci, A., and Yuce, E., "A new DVCC+ based second-order current-mode universal filter consisting of only grounded capacitors", *Journal of Circuits, Systems and Computers*, vol. 26, no. 9, 1750130, 2017.

21. Yucel, F., and Yuce, E., "Grounded capacitor based fully cascadable electronically tunable current-mode universal filter", *AEU-International Journal of Electronics and Communications*, vol. 79, pp. 116–123, 2017.

22. Yuce, E., and Minaei, S., "Universal current-mode filters and parasitic impedance effects on the filter performances", *International Journal of Circuit Theory and Applications*, vol. 36, no. 2, pp. 161–171, 2008.

23. Wang, C., Xu, J., Keskin, A. Ü., Du, S., and Zhang, Q., "A new current-mode current-controlled SIMO-type universal filter", *AEU-International Journal of Electronics and Communications*, vol. 65, no. 3, pp. 231–234, 2011.

24. Singh, S. V., Maheshwari, S., and Chauhan, D. S., "Current-processing current-controlled universal biquad filter", *Radioengineering*, vol. 21, no. 1, pp. 317–323, 2012.

25. Prommee, P., and Somdunyakanok, M., "CMOS-based current-controlled DDCC and its applications to capacitance multiplier and universal filter", *AEU-International Journal of Electronics and Communications*, vol. 65, no. 1, pp. 1–8, 2011.

26. Tangsrirat, W., "Current-tunable current-mode multifunction filter based on dual-output current-controlled conveyors", *AEU-International Journal of Electronics and Communications*, vol. 61, no. 8, pp. 528–533, 2007.

27. Siripruchyanun, M., and Jaikla, W., "Current controlled current conveyor transconductance amplifier (CCCCTA): a building block for analog signal processing", *Electrical Engineering*, vol. 90, no. 6, pp. 443–453, 2008.

28. Nand, D., and Pandey, N., "New configuration for OFCC-based CM SIMO filter and its application as shadow filter" *Arabian Journal for Science and Engineering*, vol. 43, no. 6, pp. 3011–3022, 2018.

29. Pandey, N., Nand, D., and Khan, Z., "Single-input four-output current mode filter using operational floating current conveyor", *Active and Passive Electronic Components*, vol. 2013, Article ID 318560, 2013.

30. Horng, J. W., "High output impedance current-mode universal biquadratic filters with five inputs using multi-output CCIIs", *Microelectronics Journal*, vol. 42, no. 5, pp. 693–700, 2011.

31. Horng, J. W., "Current-mode and transimpedance-mode universal biquadratic filter using multiple outputs CCIIs", *Indian Journal of Engineering and Materials Sciences*, vol. 17, no. 3, pp. 169–174, 2010.

32. Hassen, N., Ettaghzouti, T., Garradhi, K., and Besbes, K., "MISO current mode bi-quadratic filter employing high performance inverting second generation current conveyor circuit", *AEU-International Journal of Electronics and Communications*, vol. 82, pp. 191–201, 2017.

33. Kacar, F., Yesil, A., and Kuntman, H., "Current-mode biquad filters employing single FDCCII", *Radioengineering*, vol. 21, no. 4, pp. 1269–1278, 2012.

34. Singh, P., and Nagaria, R. K., "Electronically tunable DV-EXCCCII-based universal filter", *International Journal of Electronics Letters*, vol. 9, no. 3, pp. 301–317, 2020.

Chapter 8

VLSI Design and Optimization for Advanced Health Monitoring

Shipra Upadhyay
Atria Institute of Technology, Bangalore, India

Amit Kumar Pandey
Rajkiya Engineering College, Uttar Pradesh, India

Shailendra Kumar
Indian Space Research Organization, Headquarters, Bangalore, India

CONTENTS

ABBREVIATIONS

AI	Artificial Intelligence
ECG	Electro cardiograph
MATLAB	Matrix Laboratory
SOC	System on chip
VLSI	Very large scale integrated circuits

8.1 INTRODUCTION

Society is ageing at an extraordinary speed at the start of the twenty-first century. There are over 600 million individuals over the age of 60 on the globe – and also around 860 million people who are suffering from chronic diseases. Society in Asian countries is quickly growing older: the population aged 65 years old accounted for more than 23% of the population in 2010, and this is estimated to reach 30% in another six years [1]. This is followed

DOI: 10.1201/9781003431138-8

by a growth in healthcare costs, as well as in the number of people suffering from lifestyle disorders. As a result, a switch from conventional treatment to preventive medical management is urgently needed in order to improve people's standard of living and reduce medical expenses.

Experts believe that the very first step in precautionary health and medical management is to identify the patient's existing situation. Certain symptoms, such as hidden hypertension, are not revealed in the clinics; there is a strong requirement for capturing statistical information over a lengthy period of time in daily life, documenting data variation, or storing relevant data through medical observations rather than subjective data. Physicians, particularly, like to know whether the patients are following the prescribed treatment methods and diets. As a result, there is a growing demand for healthcare monitoring that can be accessed at any time and from any location. Because of developments in information and communication technology, sensors incorporated in patients' surroundings can give their health records by constantly monitoring and analyzing the patients' daily lifestyles.

This new, home-based healthcare approach has the potential to be the most cost-effective and efficient method of healthcare delivery. However, patient acceptance of this new treatment technique would be heavily reliant on user comfort and price. As an outcome, a low-power and portable sensor and transmission solution with a relatively long battery life is required for the home-based healthcare system to be successful. Furthermore, for patients being observed at home, a constant and accurate health monitoring solution is necessary. This chapter discusses a VLSI technology based single-chip solution for a wireless health monitoring system. As illustrated in Table 8.1, this provides a less costly and high-performance device with good-quality ECG signal capture and long battery life. To obtain better hand-held performance in terms of convenience and cost, the amount of off-chip components employed should be kept to a minimum. Simultaneously, low-energy and voltage operation is required for the long durability of device in constant and advanced real-time healthcare scenarios.

Table 8.1 Evolution of health monitoring system due to VLSI design advancement

Health service	Clinics, hospitals and emergency services	Home service and care	Treatment from robotic surgeries, wearable healthcare
Total cost involved	Low	Medium	High
Place of care and service	Hospitals and clinics only	Any individual's home	Anywhere as per the need
Healthcare devices	Big	Portable	Wearable (lightweight)

8.2 STUDY OF VLSI DESIGN AND OPTIMIZATION BASED ADVANCED BIOSENSING SYSTEM

During research, it was found that classifying health conditions, which include expressions such as anger, surprise and fear, is complex. This is because the natural nervous system response patterns of these emotions exhibit comparably similar ranges of arousal and valence levels. So, the major objective of this research was to classify human emotions based on EEG signals. For this purpose, an experiment was carried out among 110 students, with 57 men and 53 women between the ages of 22 and 24 years. To ensure successful outcomes from the experiment, it was ensured that the subjects did not have any history of medical illness. Linear discriminant analysis (LDA) was used to analyze the three kinds of electroencephalographic (EEG) signals and the identification accuracy was found to be 66.3%. After obtaining the LDA results, it was found that the frequency band features, cerebral asymmetry features and EEG coherence features exhibited a mean accuracy level of 57.9% 38.8% and 55.3% respectively. Therefore, the outcomes obtained from the experiment indicate that EEG signals were helpful in specifically classifying the three emotions. It can also be noted that this method can be useful when emotions need to be recognized without the utilization of facial and verbal expressions.

Another research study [2] attempted to suggest solutions for the medical consequences that can arise from the unhealthy emotions and the stress caused during day-to-day life activities. The objective of this study was to utilize the fusion EEG signals and north Indian classical music to determine the emotional stress. The music consists of various ragas and it invokes emotions in the person listening to it. During this study, the various EEG signals were extracted and their respective stimuli towards the raga was studied to interpret the emotions of the user such as happiness, anger, sadness and fear. A technique called Kernel Density Estimation was utilized to extract the EEG signal features and the emotions were interpreted using Multilayer Perceptron. The music and ragas were used to identify the stress levels and identify the emotions in the listener. The neural network classifiers exhibited better accuracy for arousal and valence models. The conclusion shows that performance of emotions during a combination of arousal and valence showed a maximum accuracy level of 95.36%, while under separate arousal and valence it showed an accuracy 91.77%. From these experiments, it was found that EEG can be considered as a reliably promising method to check and evaluate the emotions and stress levels in human beings.

As it is observed that the EEG signals effectively classify the positive and negative emotions in an individual, further research study [3] was carried out to find the relationship between human emotions and EEG signals. During this research, an experiment was carried out on three men and three women, who were all right-handed, and healthy subjects. Initially, the EEG signal features were extracted from the original extracted EEG data and a further linear dynamic system approach was used to smooth the required features. The extracted features were used with a support vector machine, which resulted in an experimental accuracy of 87.53%. Then, correlation coefficients were used to reduce the dimensions of the extracted features. This resulted in top 100 and 50 subject independent features, which resulted in an accuracy of 89.22% and 84.94%. During the final stage, a model was used to plot the trajectory of the emotional changes. It was noticed that the outcomes almost matched the true changes in emotional states. Thus, the research concludes that EEG signals-based emotion recognition and classification is a reliable methodology to detect human emotions.

This study [4] was conducted to identify the emotional states by interpreting the EEG signals generated from the EEG sensors placed at the surface of the scalp. The optimal combination of features of the extracted signals were used for recognition. The experiment was performed on 21 healthy children aged between 12 and 14 years old. A 14 channel EEG machine was used to collect the EEG signals of the subjects, which showed various response stimuli such as happiness, sadness, anger and fear. The optimal features necessary for emotional classification were processed by using a Support Vector Machine (SVM), k-nearest neighbor (KNN), Linear Discriminant Analysis (LDA), deep learning and four ensemble methods. It was further concluded that selecting optimal features is a good option for enhancing the performance during EEG-based emotion interpretation.

During another research study [5], the experiment was conducted using EEG sensors for various people. This method utilized the 10–20 international system, according to which Ag/AgCl electrodes were attached to the scalp to record the EEG signals. The amplitude and frequency of the main waves of the EEG signals such as alpha, beta, gamma and theta were checked. It was observed that the measurements were usually difficult to obtain due to smaller amplitude and large DC offset. Thus, the EEG signals were amplified using a multistage amplifier and digitized using a 24-bit analog-to-digital converter (ADC). The theoretical designs were implemented using TINA-TI software and furthermore, Eagle software was used to design, and Printed Circuit Board (PCB) for practical implementation. It was concluded that the use of EEG sensors to diagnose medical conditions prevents various aspects of patient preparation, like shaving the head, adding EEG gel to the site of electrodes and skin abrasion.

More research [6] was conducted using an 8-bit AVR RISC-based microcontroller to design and implement a filtering circuit. This research was carried out for efficient signal acquisition of EEG signals with frequencies ranging between 0.15Hz and 50Hz.This methodology is chosen since the low voltage levels of EEG signals make them hard to digitize. This study was conducted to find an alternative to substitute for the expensive ADC and Digital Signal Processors (DSPs) which were regularly used to gather and process data. Therefore, it was concluded that this research suggests a complete analog solution to record the EEG signals instead of digital filters.

Some research work [7] outcomes suggest that there are almost 66 human emotions which can be analyzed and these are further divided into two groups: basic emotions and secondary emotions.

Basic emotions can be identified more easily than secondary emotions.

8.3 VLSI DESIGN BASED ADVANCED HEALTH MONITORING SYSTEMS IN NEUROLOGICAL DISORDER CONDITIONS

Over the years, human beings and the technological world have grown dynamically. As a result, the complexity of life has also increased, leading to a dramatic rise in the number of neurological health issues such as hypertension, depression, behavioral disorders, dementia, schizophrenia and so forth. The healthcare industry has thus been utilizing multiple methods, with the help of VLSI technology [9–20, 22–37], to diagnose the aforementioned psychiatric issues. Even though facial images and voice tones are analyzed to determine the underlying complex emotions, these methods have proven to be less efficient.

Later, scientists and medical experts carried out extensive research to study the electrical activity in the brain. Although various technological advancements have occurred in the psychiatric field, this technique of analyzing brainwave patterns is considered very reliable in successfully interpreting the emotional state of an individual. The emotions are interlinked and closely associated with the healthy mental and emotional state of an individual. A better emotional condition signifies better performance; thus, emotions are thoroughly studied to understand the mental state and overall performance of human beings.

Emotion recognition and evaluation is distinguished under two categories. The initial method was conducted by analyzing non-physiological signals such as facial expressions, body language and tone of voice, while the later more advanced method was carried out by analyzing the brain's electrical activity, which is a physiological signal. Most of the earlier studies discovered and inspected human emotions based on facial expressions and voice. However, the facial expressions and voice tone of a person can be consciously controlled and modified. Thus, the methods based on non-physiological signals are unreliable. In contrast, the techniques used to measure the signals based on physiological processes in humans such as electroencephalography (EEG), electromyogram (EMG) and electrocardiogram (ECG) are clinically found to be more effective and reliable. This is because human beings cannot consciously or intentionally control the functioning of the physiological processes and the related health metrics. Among these methods, the electroencephalography-based emotion recognition technique has evolved as the most reliable and widely used technology nowadays as shown in Figure 8.1.

In this model, the EEG sensors are used to collect the brainwaves of an individual or child from the surface of their scalp, which are then further

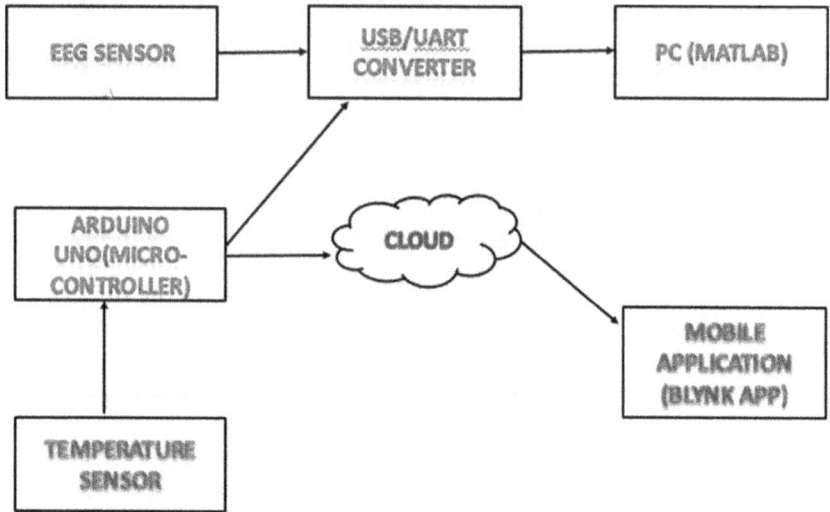

Figure 8.1 Proposed model of advanced health monitoring system.

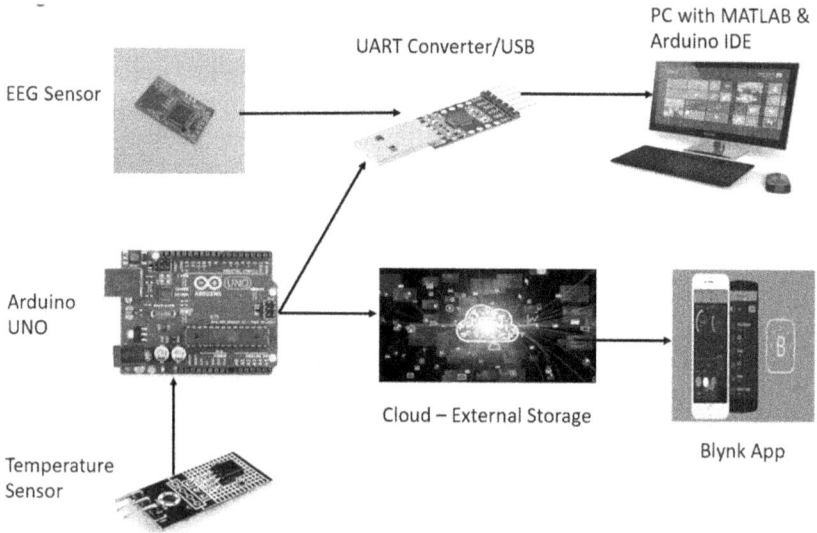

Figure 8.2 Implemented model of advanced health monitoring system.

studied. The inspection of the raw EEG brainwave signals against trained neural networks can predict the emotional or neurological state of the child or an individual. These brainwave signals are transmitted to the Arduino UNO microcontroller where the signals are processed and stored. A temperature sensor is used to check the physical health of the subject as shown in Figure 8.2.

Further, Matrix Laboratory (MATLAB) technology and signal processing techniques such as Fast Fourier Transform (FFT) or Discrete Wavelet Transform (DWT) are used to interpret the EEG signals in both the time domain and the frequency domain. In addition, certain features of the extracted EEG signals are studied against the standard frequency ranges of alpha, beta, gamma and theta. Also, these techniques assist in predicting the child's cognitive states like alert, sleepy or attentive, and emotional states like sad, happy or angry. Thus, we have successfully found an effective solution for providing necessary medical care and emergency assistance for children with mental health issues.

8.4 CONCLUSION

The healthcare industry has been utilizing multiple methods to diagnose health issues with the use of advanced VLSI design techniques. Although, in the case of emotion recognition aspects such as facial images and voice tones are analyzed to determine complex emotions, these methods have proven to be less efficient. Children prone to neurological impairments or psychiatric disorders, innately and otherwise, require real-time supervision of their mental state. In addition to that, a large number of such children are medically advised to stay at home as they lack the ability to carry out their day-to-day activities independently. Therefore, the major objective of the advanced healthcare industry is to continuously evaluate the health of the patients and further, to notify through alert messages during emergency conditions. In this chapter, we have studied various advanced health monitoring systems, such as mood swing detectors, along with an alerting system specific for emergency instances. We have also studied a hardware model built using an electroencephalography sensor and temperature sensor to inspect neurological and physical health states, and to predict the overall health of the child. Further, VLSI technology can be used for the purpose of brain-computer interfacing and signal processing. This mood swing detector supervises the electrical activity in the brain and acknowledges the cognitive functions and emotions on a real-time basis.

REFERENCES

[1] Ram K. Nawasalkar, Pradeep K. Butey, Swapnil G. Deshpande, V.M. Thakare, "EEG-Based Stress Recognition System Based on Indian Classical Music", *2015 International Conference on Advances in Computer Engineering and Applications (ICACEA)*, 23 July 2015, pp. 936–939.

[2] Mi-Sook Park, Hyeong-Seok Dh, Hoyeon Jeong, Jin-Hun Sohn, Department of Psychology, Brain Research Institute, Chungnam National University, Daejeon, S. Korea, "EEG-based Emotion Recognition during Emotionally Evocative

Films", *2013 International Winter Workshop on Brain-Computer Interface (BCI)*, 23 April 2013, pp. 56–57.

[3] Dan Nie, Xiao-Wei Wang, Li-Chen Shi, and Bao-Liang Lu Senior Member, IEEE, "EEG-Based Emotion Recognition during Watching Movies", *International IEEE EMBS Conference on Neural Engineering Cancun*, Mexico, April 27–May 1, 2011, pp. 667–670.

[4] Raja Majid Mehmood, Ruoyu Du, Hyo Jong Lee, "Optimal feature selection and Deep Learning Ensembles Method for emotion recognition from human brain EEG sensors", *IEEE Access* 31 July 2017, vol. 5, pp. 14797–14806.

[5] Safaa Saod Mahdi, Mahir Rahman Al-Hajaj "Design and Implementation of EEG Measuring System". *The First National Conference for Engineering Sciences FNCES'12* / November 7–8, 2012, pp. 1–3.

[6] Jose Perez, Jimmy Tarrillo "Implementation of an Active-Filtering Circuit for Electroencephalographic Signal Acquisition Using an 8-bit Microcontroller". *2020 IEEE 14th Dallas Circuits and Systems Conference (DCAS)*, 25 January 2021.

[7] Dzedzickis A, Kaklauskas A, Bucinskas V. Human Emotion Recognition: Review of Sensors and Methods. Sensors (Basel) 2020 Jan 21;20(3):592. doi: 10.3390/s20030592.

[8] Muneer, Amgad, and Suliman Mohamed Fati. "Automated Health Monitoring System Using Advanced Technology," Journal of Information Technology Research (JITR) 12, no.3: 104–132. http://doi.org/10.4018/JITR.2019070107

[9] T. H. Teo et al., "A 700-μ W Wireless Sensor Node SoC for Continuous Real-Time Health Monitoring," in IEEE Journal of Solid-State Circuits, vol. 45, no. 11, pp. 2292–2299, Nov. 2010, doi: 10.1109/JSSC.2010.2064030.

[10] Bluetooth SIG, "Health Device Profile Specification Vol. 1.0," http://www.bluetooth.org/

[11] Continua Health Alliance, "Version2010 Design Guidelines," http://www.continuaalliance.org/products/design-guidelines.html

[12] JST (Japan Science and Technology Agency)–CREST (Core Research for Evolutional Science & Technology) project on, "Development of a Physiological and Environmental Information Processing Platform and its Application to the Metabolic Syndrome Measures," http://www.jst.go.jp/kisoken/crest/en/area02/1-01.html

[13] M. Shuzo, and I. Yamada, "Development of Biological & Environmental Information Processing Platform," in *Proceedings of the 2009 Japan Electrical Engineering Society Technical Meeting*, Sapporo, March 2009 (in Japanese).

[14] J. Espina, T. Falck, J. Muehlsteff, Y. Jin, M. A. Adan, and X. Aubert, "Wearable Body Sensor Network Towards Continuous Cuff-less Blood Pressure Monitoring," *Proceedings of the 5th International Summer School and Symposium on Medical Devices and Biosensors (ISSS-MDBS 2008)*, pp. 28–32, 2008.

[15] D. McCombie, A. Reisner, and H. Asada, "Motion-based Adaptive Calibration of Pulse Transit Time Measurements to Arterial Blood Pressure for an Autonomous, Wearable Blood Pressure Monitor," *Proceedings of the 30th Annual International Conference of the IEEE Engineering in Medicine and Biology Society (EMBC 2008)*, pp. 989–992, 2008.

[16] G. Lopez, M. Shuzo, H. Ushida, K. Hidaka, S. Yanagimoto, Y. Imai, A. Kosaka, J.-J. Delaunay, and I. Yamada, "Continuous Blood Pressure Monitoring in Daily Life,"

Journal of Advanced Mechanical Design, Systems, and Manufacturing, vol. 4, no. 1, pp. 179–186, 2010, http://www.nittokagaku.com/kamikami/product. html

[17] J. Nishimura, and T. Kuroda, "Eating Habits Monitoring Using Wireless Wearable In-Ear Microphone," in *Proceedings of International Symposium on Wireless Pervasive Communications (ISWPC08)*, IEEE, 2008.

[18] H. Zhang, G. Lopez, M. Shuzo, J.-J. Delaunay, and I. Yamada, "Mastication Counting Method Robust to Food Type and Individual," *International Conference on Health Informatics (HEALTHINF 2012)*, pp. 374–377, 2012.

[19] H. Zhang, G. Lopez, R. Tao, M. Shuzo, J.-J. Delaunay, and I. Yamada, "Food Texture Estimation from Chewing Sound Analysis," *International Conference on Health Informatics (HEALTHINF 2012)*, pp. 213–218, 2012.

[20] C. Schubert, M. Lambertz, and R. Nelesen, "Effects of Stress on Heart Rate Complexity – A Comparison Between Short-Term and Chronic Stress," *Biological Psychology*, vol. 80, no. 3, pp. 325–332, 2009.

[22] K. Itao, T. Umeda, G. Lopez, and M. Kinjo, "Human Recorder System Development for Sensing the Autonomic Nervous System," *Proceedings of the 7th Annual IEEE Conference on Sensors (Sensors 2008)*, pp. 423–426, October 2008.

[23] S. Miyake, "Factors Influencing Mental Workload Indexes," *Journal of University of Occupational and Environmental Health (J. UOEH)*, vol. 19, no. 4, pp. 313–325, 1997.

[24] S. Miyake, "Multivariate Workload Evaluation Combining Physiological and Subjective Measures," *International Journal of Psychophysiology*, vol. 40, no. 3, pp. 233–238, 2001.

[25] A. Sul, J. Shin, C. Lee, Y. Yoon, and J. Principe, "Evaluation of Stress Reactivity and Recovery Using Biosignals and Fuzzy Theory," *Proceedings of the 2nd Joint EMBS-BMES Conference*, pp. 32–33, 2002.

[26] H. Ide, G. Lopez, M. Shuzo, S. Mitsuyoshi, J.-J. Delaunay, and I. Yamada, "Workplace Stress Estimation Method Based on Multivariate Analysis of Physiological Indices," *International Conference on Health Informatics (HEALTHINF 2012)*, pp. 53–60, 2012.

[27] Young-Jin Cha, Yeesock Kim, Taesun You, "Advanced Sensing and Structural Health Monitoring", *Journal of Sensors*, vol. 2018, Article ID 7286069, 3 pages, 2018. https://doi.org/10.1155/2018/7286069.

[28] Shipra Upadhyay, R. K. Nagaria and R. A. Mishra, "Complementary Energy Path Adiabatic Logic based Full Adder Circuit", *A Journal of World Academy of Science Engineering & Technology (WASET)*,vol. 66, pp.161–167, 2012.

[29] Shipra Upadhyay, R.A. Mishra and R.K. Nagaria, "DFAL: Diode Free Adiabatic Logic Circuits", *International Scholarly Research Network: ISRN Electronics, Hindawi Publishing Corporation*, vol. 2013, Article ID 673601, pp. 1–12, 2013.

[30] Shipra Upadhyay, R. K. Nagaria and R. A. Mishra, "Low-Power Adiabatic Computing with Improved Quasi Static Energy Recovery Logic", *VLSI Design*, vol. 2013, Article ID 726324, pp. 1–9.

[31] Shipra Upadhyay, R. A. Mishra, R. K. Nagaria et al. "Triangular Power Supply Based Adiabatic Logic Circuits", *World Applied Sciences Journal (WASJ)*, *IDOSI Publications*, vol. 24, no. 4, pp. 444–450, Aug. 2013.

[32] Shipra Upadhyay, R. K. Nagaria and R. A. Mishra, "Performance Improvement of GFCAL Circuits", *International Journal of Computer Applications*, vol. 78, no. 5, pp. 29–37, Sept. 2013.

[33] Shipra Upadhyay, R.A. Mishra, and R.K. Nagaria, "Performance Analysis of Modified QSERL Circuit", *International Journal of VLSI design & Communication Systems (VLSICS)*, vol. 4, no. 4, pp. 19–30, Aug. 2013.

[34] Vishnu S, Abhisheka, Anilkumar J. B., Dhanush M and Shipra Upadhyay, "Intelligent Food Distribution Sysytem", *International journal of Engineering Research in Electronics and Communication Engineering (IJERECE)*, vol. 4, no. 6, pp. 296–299, June 2017.

[35] Amit Kumar Pandey, Shipra Upadhyay, Tarun Kumar Gupta, and Pawan Kumar Verma. "Low Power, High Speed and Noise Immune Wide-OR Footless Domino Circuit Using Keeper-Controlled Method." Analog Integrated Circuits and Signal Processing, vol. 100, issue 1, pp. 79–91, July 2019. Springer US.

[36] Shipra Upadhyay, Amit Kumar Pandey and Shailendra Kumar, "Performance Evaluation of Low Power Adiabatic Techniques", TEST engineering & management, vol. 82, pp. 4132–4137, Jan 2020.

[37] Shipra Upadhyay, Amit Kumar Pandey, Shailendra Kumar Pandey, Tarun Gupta, Digvijay Pandey "Investigation of Power on Silicon Adiabatic for VLSI Applications", Silicon, no. 1615, Jan. 2022, Springer.

Chapter 9

Neural Interfacing and Monitoring by Integrated Circuit

Vinay Kumar and Chetna Bisht

Graphic Era (deemed to be a university), Uttarakhand, India

CONTENTS

ABBREVIATIONS

CFM	Carbon fiber microelectrode
CVD	Chemical vapor deposition
FET	Field effect transistor
FSCV	Fast-scan cyclic voltammetry
HRTEM	High resolution transmission electron microscopy
IDE	Interdigitated electrodes
MWCNTs	Multi-walled carbon nanotubes

9.1 INTRODUCTION

Rapid communication over long distances within the nervous system is made possible by action potentials that are transported through the neuronal axon to the synapse. A synapse is the point of contact between two neurons; basically, the transmission of information takes place here, at this contact point. Most synapses are formed between axons and dendrites. So, this is also known as the junction points of two neurons. However, the release and absorption of neurotransmitters at the intersection point between two neurons mediates communication [1, 2]. As depicted in Figure 9.1, the action potential causes the release of neurotransmitters from the pre-synaptic neuron, which diffuses towards the post-synaptic neuron and binds to certain protein receptors.

DOI: 10.1201/9781003431138-9

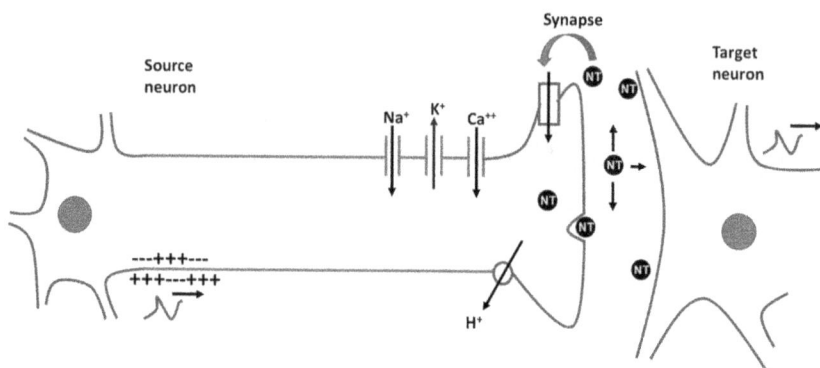

Figure 9.1 Schematic for neuronal signaling.

Pre-synaptic neurons and post-synaptic neurons are biological signal transmitters in the human body. The incoming signal of the synapse is transmitted by the pre-synaptic neuron, and the outgoing signals of the synapse by the post-synaptic neurons. Whether a new action potential will be produced ultimately depends on this change in the target neuron's physiological state.

Numerous neurological diseases, like Parkinson's disease and Alzheimer's as well as epilepsy, have been related to abnormal fluctuations in the neurotransmitter's physiological levels within the brain [3]. Numerous neuroactive chemicals, including prescription medications and illicit narcotics, work by altering the amounts of neurotransmitters at synapses or by simulating those neurotransmitters' effects at post-synaptic receptors. Additionally, changes to chemical synapses are largely responsible for the nervous system's plasticity, which supports memory and learning. Numerous aminergic systems related to biogenic, such as those that produce serotonin or dopamine, deliver responses to significant brain areas that influence mood, cognition and learning [4]. As a result, to provide a more complete picture of the neuro-signal pathways, both chemical and electrical activity measurements are needed.

9.2 CHEMICAL MONITORING

Although alternative approaches with imaging technologies in the medical field of optical probes have also been employed, microdialysis and voltammetry still dominate the field of neurochemical monitoring [5, 6]. Voltammetry and microdialysis both have unique monitoring advantages [7, 8]. Since a sample is actually extracted from the brain with the help of a probe, microdialysis of the sample can be combined with extremely sensitive and specific analytical techniques including electrophoresis, chromatography, mass spectrometry and fluorescence detection. Fluorescence detection is a kind of optical detection in which samples are tested with UV-viz spectroscopy and photoluminescence spectroscopy. Both of these types of spectroscopy examine the optical behavior of the samples, like bandgap and optical excitation emission. For detection of emission properties of the samples, first the samples are examined via UV-viz spectroscopy, from where we can get the optical absorption wavelength of the sample. Thereafter, the samples are tested for photoluminescence spectroscopy. In this study, first samples get excited by a wavelength (known as excitation wavelength) near the absorption wavelength obtained from UV-viz study, then, after excitation with a particular wavelength, we get the optical emission wavelength of the samples. This emission wavelength can be compared with standard emission wavelength of the normal sample.

In contrast, voltammetry is excellent at making rapid measurements with small probes and can easily find neurotransmitters in the brain that are present electrochemically. With the energy for the electron transfer being provided by the applied electrode potential, electrochemistry is the act of transferring charges in both directions between an electrode and a sample that is either liquid or solid [9]. Chemical reactions occur inside the probed sample volume at the surface of the electrode or very near it, and the resulting charge transfer or current – which is proportional to the electroactive neurotransmitter's concentration – is then used to determine the concentration. Dopamine, serotonin, norepinephrine, nitric oxide, and histamine are only a few significant neurotransmitters that can be detected electrochemically since they are electroactive [10]. Additionally, wireless devices can contain voltammetry [11]. Voltammetry is the greatest option for chemical measurements due to these characteristics.

Amperometry is the process of measuring current at contact points when voltage is applied [12] – it's a kind of electroanalytical process; high-speed chronoamperometry is the stepping process of a working electrode's potential via electrochemical analysis [13]; and fast-scan cyclic voltammetry (FSCV) techniques used for neurotransmission in the human brain [14]. These are the three voltammetric techniques that are currently most frequently used. Despite the fact that each carbon fiber microelectrode (CFM) monitors, an analyte having a sub-second of temporal resolution, performance variations have led to various applications in the field of cell biology and neurology systems [15]. The highest level of specificity is offered by FSCV, which is regarded as the best method for intensive care of endogenous neurotransmitters in behavioral animals since it records a chemical signature known as a cyclic voltammogram and is a powerful tool to examine the oxidation and reduction process of species in molecular level. It works on the principle of electrochemical analysis to identify the discovered species.

9.3 SENSING TECHNOLOGY AND CIRCUIT

9.3.1 Sensing Probes for Neurochemical Detection

Microelectrodes using carbon fiber, gold electrodes and micro-fabricated screen-printed polymer carbon sensors for the electrochemical detection of neurotransmitters [16, 17] have all been used by researchers in the past. Traditional neurochemical sensing probes, called carbon-fiber microelectrodes (CFMs), allow for the oxidizable species generated by individual cells and vesicles to be detected directly and with extreme sensitivity [17]. These electrodes are normally created by drawing a regular pipette puller to taper a single carbon fiber having diameter in the range of 5–10μm into a capillary tube made up of borosilicate glass. Under a microscope, the uncovered carbon fiber is then chopped to the desired length (usually between 100 and 250μm). Then, a lead wire made of stainless steel is placed into the capillary's open end and attached to the carbon fiber and glass capillary using graphite powder or molten bismuth.

A potential superior electrode biomaterial emerging nowadays is conductive Multi-Walled Carbon Nanotubes (MWCNTs). Their low baseline current and chemical and mechanical robustness enable long-term use and higher sensitivity for detecting lower analyte concentrations. MWCNTs broad window of water stability allows for the research of new chemistries. Additionally, adsorption and oxygen reduction are discouraged by the MWCNTs known surface chemistry.

The fabrication of these MWCNTs for electrodes involves employing thermal chemical vapor deposition (CVD) to selectively deposit highly conductive, boron-doped MWCNTs onto the polished surface of interdigitated microelectrodes, as shown in Figure 9.2. The high resolution transmission electron microscopy (HRTEM) image of the MWCNTs deposited over the interdigitated electrodes (IDEs) is also shown on the upper side of Figure 9.2. We can easily see the structure and lattices of the MWCNTs in this figure.

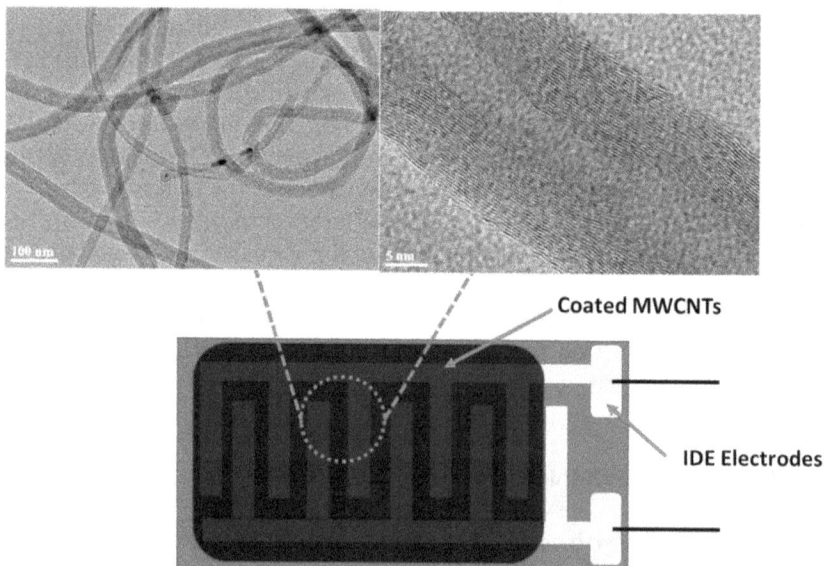

Figure 9.2 HRTEM images of MWCNTs deposited on a tungsten interdigitated microelectrode.

The fabrication of MWCNTs nanosheet-based sensing devices will be attempted in two ways. In the first scheme, field effect transistor (FET) devices will be fabricated using as prepared MWCNTs nanosheet. The traditional photolithography technique will be used for the fabrication of the source and drain electrodes of MWCNTs nanosheets as gate-based FET devices. The channel length for all FET devices will be kept in the micrometer range (about 3μm). For patterning, the source and the drain electrodes 50nm Au will be deposited by the electron beam evaporator and the photoresist will be removed thereafter.

In the second method, the tungsten/gold fabricated inter-digitated electrodes (IDEs) will be patterned on the substrate (SiO2) using photolithography and metal deposition technique. Different steps are required to develop this pattern. The first step is cleaning the SiO2 wafers using ultrasonication in acetone or methanol, and next the IDEs and the contact pads will be developed using a photoresist. A thin layer (nm) of Cr/Au/W will be deposited on the wafer using an electron beam evaporation technique. The layer of photoresist will be removed via ultrasonication in acetone. The dimensions of the developed IDEs will be 10μm × 100μm in width and length of the strip, the inter-digitated gap between the corresponding two strips is fixed as 5μm to get the desired IDEs. The fabricated IDEs will be used for electrical and sensing measurements using a Keithley 4200 semiconductor characterization system. A network of the MWCNTs nanosheet will be deposited on the fabricated IDEs.

A tungsten microstrip with dimensions 10μm × 100μm × 5μm (width × length × gap) is pre-sealed into a silicon substrate to create the microelectrode substrates. In a typical acetylene/argon/trimethylboron CVD environment, MWCNTs are preferentially deposited for up to 20 minutes at 850°C. These MWCNTs-coated interdigitated microelectrodes resemble the unique surface geometry of commercially available carbon- and metal-based (like tungsten, gold, silver, platinum, etc.) microelectrodes. As a result, it allows for insertion with little tissue injury and, when utilized in fast-scan mode, allows kinetic studies to proceed without being impacted by mass transfer issues. Using MWCNT electrodes, biogenic amines have been electrochemically identified in vitro at millisecond time periods, for example, serotonin, close to specific, recognized nerve cells in a sea snail named *Aplysia California*.

9.3.2 Interface Circuitry for Neurochemical Sensing

A neurophysiological application's potential exposure to a wide range of input currents is the key issue in integrated interface electronics design for electrochemically based neurochemistry. These currents may require resolution levels as low as a few pA, but they may also approach hundreds of nA. Because physiological neurotransmitter concentration levels do not change significantly over time, delta-sigma ($\Delta\Sigma$) represents the front-end architectures that allow a trade-off between resolution and conversion speed that are most suitable for the detection of current signals having very low-frequencies, that result from electrochemical transduction. Previous investigations for amperometric biosensors are used to detect the signal generated by the oxidation or reduction in biological elements that provides the signal to analyze the quantitative information, that has been reported using single-channel integrated circuits and multi-channel integrated circuits for interfacing, some of which use a first-order $\Delta\Sigma$ modulator ($\Delta\Sigma$ M) front-end architecture.

The architecture of a wireless monitoring system is depicted in Figure 9.3, which includes both external receiver electronics and an implantable integrated transmitter chip. When set up for neurochemistry, the chip can handle FSCV and amperometry. The sensing electrode is connected to a reconfigurable third-order M on the transmitter side, which can measure electrophysiological voltages or electric currents inversely proportional to fluctuations in extracellular concentrations of neurotransmitter levels. After on-chip Manchester encoding, the M's bit-stream for digital output is wirelessly broadcast to the outside via a back-end radio frequency-frequency shift keying (RF-FSK) transmitter. This transmitter is used to transmit the digitally encoded data in binary form; these have two states –0 and 1 FSK mechanism. In the neurochemical sensing mode, a standard chloridized silver wire (AgCl/Ag) serving as the reference electrode receives the FSCV scanning waveform from an on-chip arbitrary waveform generator. Because many neurotransmitters have physiological concentrations that are on the nanomolar range, electrochemical detection of neurotransmitters typically involves very tiny currents. The ohmic drop across the reference electrode would be minimal as a result. With no counter electrode required, a two-electrode electro-analysis device can be used.

The core recording module, as depicted in Figure 9.4, is a third-order continuous-time $\Delta\Sigma M$ with a single-bit quantizer. A single-bit quantizer is a

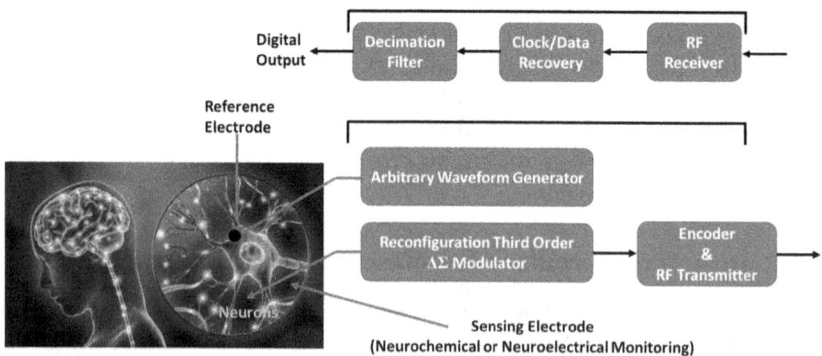

Figure 9.3 The single-channel integrated circuit's architectural design allows for wireless monitoring of cerebral activity, either chemical or electrical. When set up for neurochemistry, the chip may accommodate FSCV and amperometry.

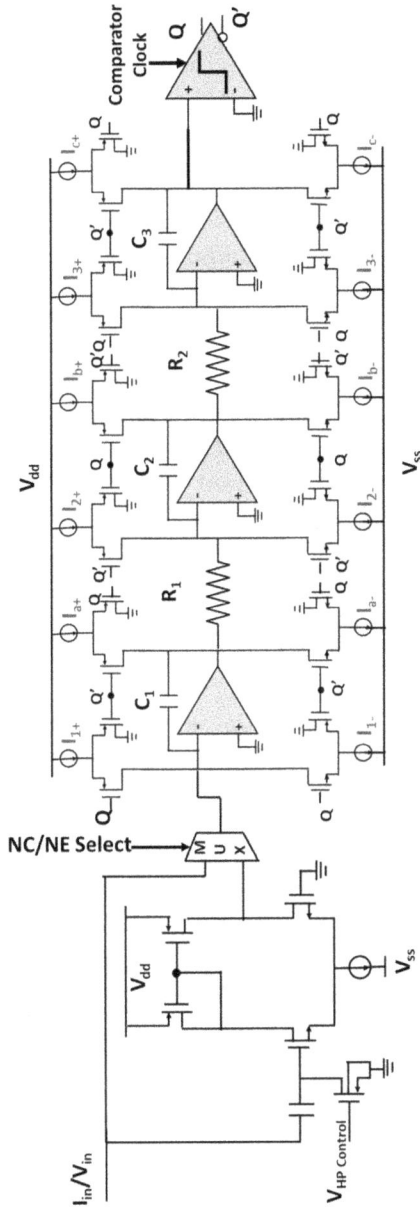

Figure 9.4 Circuit diagram for the primary sensing element, which comprises a third order current-input single-bit quantization (ΔΣM) and a front-end V/I converter with dc baseline stabilization.

device in which a large set of data can be quantized in a countable set of digital data. Its silicon area is 850μm × 180μm, and when it is clocked at 680kHz, it wastes 28μA from a 2.5V supply. For very low current sensing applications, amplification of the current is required to avoid intrinsic noise and nonlinearity, as it consistently translates incredibly small currents into digital data. It is made to be stable in the 750nA targeted input range needed for FSCV neurochemical detection.

The integrating amplifiers are required for slew rate and bandwidth also to relax these parameters. Like slew rate and bandwidth, the sets of current sources (I_a, I_b, and I_c) are additionally required, too, resulting in the current usage of only 4.4μA per amplifier. The slew rate of an integrated amplifier is the optimum change in the rate of the output voltage of the amplifier; it measures in voltage per microsecond (V/μs). I_1, I_2, and I_3 make up the majority of the source pairs from feedback current for the ΔΣM addition or subtraction.

A block that transforms controlled currents from neuroelectrical input voltages in the V range using ac coupling, and open loop transconductance (Gm) by the ΔΣM for further processing, can also be used to set up the recording channel for electrophysiological experiments. The Gm block uses a silicon area of 100μm × 180μm, draws about 3.6μA, and includes a sub-threshold P-channel metal oxide semiconductor (PMOS) transistor and a 4-pF on-chip capacitor (Cin) for dc baseline stabilization.

REFERENCES

[1] M.J. Zigmond, F.E. Bloom, S.C. Landis, J.L. Roberts, and L.R. Squire (1999) *Fundamental Neuroscience*. San Diego: Academic Press.

[2] E.R. Kandel, J.H. Schwartz, and T.M. Jessell (2000) *Principles of Neural Science*. New York: McGraw-Hill.

[3] Lei Wang, Jie Shen, Xin-Ting Cai, Wei-Wei Tao, Ya-Di Wan, Dong-Lin Li, Xiu-Xiu Tan, Yu Wang, "Ventrolateral periaqueductal gray matter neurochemical lesion facilitates epileptogenesis and enhances pain sensitivity in epileptic rats", *Neuroscience*, vol. 411, 105–118, 2019.

[4] M.E. Hasselmo, J. Hay, M. Ilyn, and A. Gorchetchnikov, "Neuromodulation, theta rhythm and rat spatial navigation", *Neural Networks*, vol. 15, pp. 689–707, 2002.

[5] Mengjie Qie, Shuangyue Li, Chuntao Guo, Shuming Yang, Yan Zhao, "Study of the occurrence of toxic alkaloids in forage grass by liquid chromatography tandem mass spectrometry", *Journal of Chromatography A*, vol. 1654, 462463, 2021.

[6] J. Mercier, L. Provins, J. Hannestad, "Progress and challenges in the development of PET ligands to aid CNS drug discovery", *Comprehensive Medicinal Chemistry*, vol. III, 20–65, 2017.

[7] P.E.M. Phillips and R.M. Wightman, "Critical guidelines for validation of the selectivity of in vivo chemical microsensors". *Trends in Analytical Chemistry*, vol. 22, 509–514, 2003.

[8] C.J. Watson, B.J. Venton, and R.T. Kennedy, "In vivo measurements of neurotransmitters by microdialysis sampling". *Analytical Chemistry*, vol. 78, 1391–1399, 2006.

[9] K. S. Demirci, L. A. Beardslee, S. Truax, J.-J. Su, O. Brand, "Integrated silicon-based chemical microsystem for portable sensing applications", *Sensors and Actuators B: Chemical*, vol. 180, 50–59, 2013.

[10] L.M. Borland and A.C. Michael (2007) "An introduction to electrochemical methods in neuroscience". In: *Electrochemical Methods for Neuroscience* (Michael AC, Borland LM, eds), Boca Raton: CRC Press, 1–15, 2007.

[11] P.A. Garris, P.G. Greco, S.G. Sandberg, G. Howes, S. Pongmayteegul, B.A. Heidenreich, J.M. Casto, R. Ensman, J. Poehlman, A. Alexander, and G.V. Rebec, "In vivo voltam- metry with telemetry". In: *Electrochemical Methods for Neuroscience*, Boca Raton: CRC Press, 233–259, 2006.

[12] F. Gonon, "Monitoring dopamine and noradrenaline release in central and peripheral nervous systems with treated and untreated carbon-fiber electrodes". In: Boulton, A.A., Baker, G.B., Adams, R.N. (eds) *Neuromethods: Voltammetric Methods in Brain Systems*, vol. 27, Totowa, New Jersey: Humana Press, 153–177, 1995.

[13] Wenhu Yang, Hao Guo, Rui Xue, Xin Zhao, Qixia Guan, Tian Fan, Longwen Zhang, Fan Yang, Wu Yang, "0.2CNT/NiSex composite derived from CNT/MOF-74 as electrode material for electrochemical capacitor and electrochemical sensor", *Microchemical Journal*, vol. 168, 106519, 2021.

[14] Jordan T. Lloyd, Andrew G. Yee, Prasanna K. Kalligappa, Anower Jabed, Pang Y. Cheung, Kathryn L. Todd, Rashika N. Karunasinghe, Srdjan M. Vlajkovic, Peter S. Freestone, Janusz Lipski, "Dopamine dysregulation and altered responses to drugs affecting dopaminergic transmission in a new dopamine transporter knockout (DAT-KO) rat model", *Neuroscience*, vol. 491, 43–64, 2022.

[15] S.G. Sandberg and P.A. Garris, "Neurochemistry of addiction: monitoring essential neurotransmitter of addiction". In: Kuhn CM, Koob GF, (eds). *Advances in the Neuroscience of Addiction.*, Boca Raton: CRC Press, 2007.

[16] M. Naware, N.V. Thakor, R.N. Orth, K. Murari, and P.A. Passeraub, "Design and microfabrication of a polymer-modified carbon sensor array for the measurement of neurotransmitter signals", in *Proc. 25th Annu. Int. IEEE Eng. Med. Biol. Conf. (EMBC'03), 1952–1955*, Cancun, Mexico, 2003.

[17] P.S. Cahill, Q.D. Walker, J.M. Finnegan, G.E. Mickelson, and R.M. Wightman, "Microelectrodes for the measurement of catecholamines in biological systems", *Analytical Chemistry*, vol. 68, 3180–3186, 1996.

Chapter 10

Applications of Nanobiosensors for Biomedical and Healthcare Monitoring Systems

A Review and Prospective Study

Akanksha Gupta
United Institute of Pharmacy, Prayagraj, India

Abhinav Gupta
Rajkiya Engineering College Sonbhadra, Sonbhadra, Uttar Pradesh, India

Vikrant Varshney
Electronic Design Automation Group (EDAG), Circuit Design & TCAD Solutions, Synopsys (India) Pvt. Ltd., India

Anurag Sewak
Rajkiya Engineering College Sonbhadra, Sonbhadra, Uttar Pradesh, India

CONTENTS

ABBREVIATIONS

CNT	Carbon nanotubes
FET	Field effect transistor
GNPs	Gold nanoparticles
IC	Integrated circuit
IUPAC	International Union of Pure and Applied Chemistry
MNP	Magnetic nanoparticles
MWCNT	Multi-walled carbon nanotubes
NiNPs	Nickel hexa-cyanoferrate nanoparticles

DOI: 10.1201/9781003431138-10

NP	Nanoparticles
PDMS	Polydimethylsiloxane
PET	Polyethylene terephthalate
QD	Quantum dot
SWCNTs	Single-walled carbon nanotubes

10.1 INTRODUCTION

A sensor is an electronic device through which we can sense various aspects such as chemicals, biology, temperatures, mechanical motions, electricity, magnetics, electromagnetics, optics and others [1]. Nanotechnology will augment the performance of sensors with a convinced impression on the development and growth of novel biosensors [2]. In the recent era of advanced nanotechnology, biosensing gadgets are developed to fulfil the demand of many areas including the defense forces, medical science, biotechnology and earth sciences [3].

Scientists and researchers are working in collaboration to develop highly reliable biosensors to perform significantly [4]. By the end of 2022, the extent of wearable biosensing devices will reach above 1 billion worldwide [5]. Improving the healthcare and telemedicine systems with continuous advancement in technology has gained the attention of engineers in both the diagnostic as well as therapeutic fields. Recently, wireless telemonitoring has been developed as a possible alternative technology in the field of biomedical and healthcare systems [6].

A biosensor is a gadget which consists of a bio-element, a transducer and a detector unit [7]. The bio-elements are produced by biological technology and comprise various cell tissues, enzymes, cell receptors, microbes and so on [8]. The transducer is a component which converts one form of energy to another form of energy. It interacts with the bio-element and can normally evaluate, as well as define, the interaction of analyte in the form of optical, electromagnetics, piezoelectric or electrochemical signal [9]. By means of a transducing mechanism, feedback on the bio-element is converted into a distinct and reproducible form [10]. It has become a bottleneck for scientists to develop an effective biosensor with low cost and complexity [11].

10.2 CATEGORIES OF BIOSENSORS

A novel biosensor has been developed with a nanomaterial which is capable of detecting chemical and biological molecules. It is basically a mixture of biosensing elements, inorganic, organic or hybrid nanoparticles. Nanomaterials such as semiconductors, nanotubes, field effect transistors (FET), carbon nanotubes (CNT) and so on, having various kinds of structure and shapes, can be used for designing biosensors. Something which can distinguish a chemical compound, mainly with the help of thermal, electrical or optical signals, can be termed as a biosensor as per International Union of Pure and Applied Chemistry (IUPAC). It consists of a significant biochemical reaction facilitated by an isolated enzyme, tissue or whole cell [12]. The nanoparticles are fabricated above the wafer surface and this is in absolute connection with that of biological sensing elements. The most appropriate materials for designing biosensors are carbon nanotubes, silicon nanowires, graphene and conducting polymer tubes [13]. Through integrated circuit (IC) technology, the operation of biosensors can be greatly enhanced [14]. The most appropriate device for osseo-integration of a bone implant is a titanium implant as it can remain infection free. To assess the osseo-integration with the bone cells, ultrasonic elastic guided waves are used [15]. To fabricate highly scalable, low-cost flexible sensors, carbon nanomaterials are used [16]. In recent years, biomaterial-based pH sensors have been used for osseo-integrated tissue prostheses interface. Transition metal oxides such as TiO_2, Co_3O_4, NiO, and CuO exhibit excellent stability and high sensitivity. Hence, these are significantly used to develop electrochemical glucose biosensors. Advanced 2D materials, such as MoS_2, have emerged as potential materials for the preparation of bioabsorbable sensors [17].

For continuous monitoring of patient health and to monitor the progression of disease, it is crucial to quantify the stress in tissues such as blood vessels, brain, eyes and bladder [18]. Hence, it becomes quite complex to take periodic and accurate measurement of stress in order to define the treatment protocol that can reduce the proportion of injury and augment the proportion of recovery. After a predetermined interval, the component material of bioresorbable sensors dissolve in the bio fluid. Consequently, the requirement for the clinical elimination of sensing devices after scientific use has been eliminated with bioresorbable sensors. Both doctors and patients are forced toward electronic and mobile healthcare due to the advancement in the modern biomedical and healthcare systems [19]. To remotely monitor the health of patients, smart wearable body sensors are employed. These sensors provide all necessary information about the disease which helps doctors to treat the disease accurately and precisely with the help of a continuous monitoring system. These sensing elements are proficient in computing variables and direct the information either to a personal device or to an online databank. Thus, they can be effective diagnostic tools for the detection and treatment of various diseases.

In electrochemical biosensors, the response of the biosensing part is transformed into an electrical equivalent signal by a transducer, whose amplitude depends on the concentration of specific analyte. Figure 10.1 shows the schematic diagram of an electrochemical biosensor. It can be classified as a biocatalytic biosensor and affinity biosensor. The biocatalytic biosensor responds with a specific analyte to tissues, enzymes or cells. Whereas affinity biosensors work on the basis of selective binding interaction between the biosensing element and analyte. Due to metabolic illness, shortage of insulin and hyperglycemia, diabetes may occur in a patient. It can be deemed as a

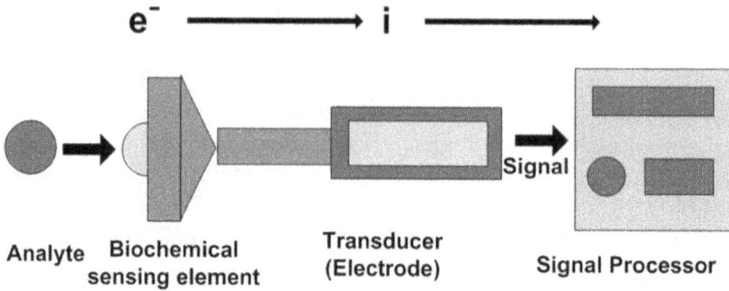

Figure 10.1 Diagram of an electrochemical biosensor.

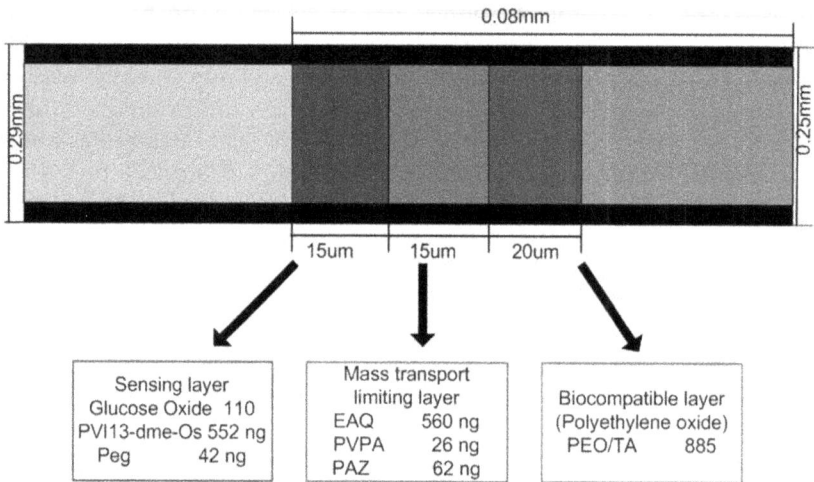

Figure 10.2 Diagram of an implantable glucose biosensor.

universal health problem. There is a chance of kidney failure, blindness or heart failure, if a patient exhibits a lower or higher glucose level concentration than that of the standard span of 80–120mg/dL [20]. Hence, it is important to continuously monitor the glucose level of a patient to monitor and maintain their health. Figure 10.2 shows the block diagram of an implantable glucose biosensor.

Field-effect transistor (FET) biosensors are receiving the interest of researchers with the advancement of novel nanomaterials and nanofabrication facilities. The main advantage of using FET biosensors is their facility of direct transforming of the communication of target biomolecules into electrical signals. The biosensing molecules are placed near the semiconductor channel and the channel will directly interact with the target biomolecules in a FET biosensor [21]. Figure 10.3 shows a dielectric modulated FET biosensor [22] in which the biomolecules modulate the gate oxide permittivity due to targeted molecules. This will cause an alteration in the

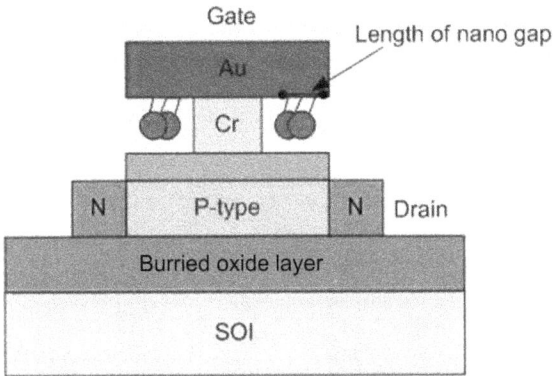

Figure 10.3 Dielectric modulated FET biosensor [21].

drain current of the FET biosensor. This change in the drain current will help in observing the healthiness of a patient. These biosensors can be employed to identify biotin and are proficient at sensing biomolecules such as cancer-markers, DNA and antibodies. The size of biomolecules and carbon nanotubes are approximately the same; due to this, the biosensor is capable of detecting single molecular events. Figure 10.4 shows a single walled carbon nanotube FET biosensor employing a Polydimethylsiloxane

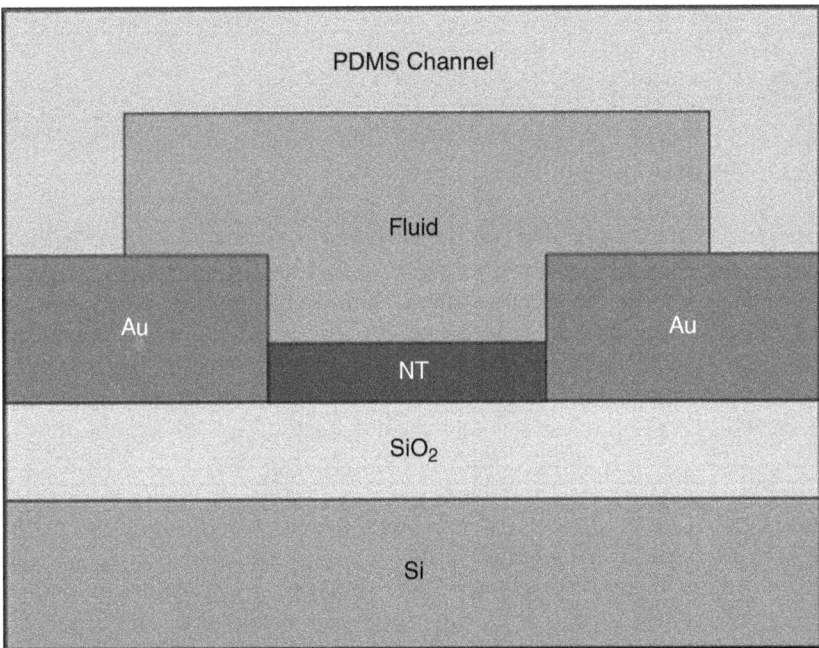

Figure 10.4 Single-walled CNT FET biosensor [22].

Table 10.1 Classification of biosensors

Type of biosensor	Materials used	Application
Bioresorbable	1. SiO$_2$ and Si 2. Zn, Mg, Mo, Fe, MgO, silk, SiN$_x$, polylactic-coglycolic acid, polylactic acid and oly-caprolactone	1. Pressure recognition 2. Temperature identifying
Flexible and wearable	1. Zinc, tin, platinum and nickel 2. Polyethylene terephthalate (PET), polycarbonate and polyurethane	1. Observing of neurological function 2. Physical therapy and Rehabilitation 3. Vascular & cardiopulmonary observing 4. Glucose checking
Electrochemical	1. Oxidase, glucose, nanomembranes and nanowires 2. Carbon nanotube	1. Glucose recognition, humidity distinguishing 2. Recognition of homo-cysteine-biomarker
Field Effect Transistor	1. SiO$_2$ and Si 2. Semiconductor materials 3. Carbon nanotube 4. MoS$_2$	1. Recognition of biotin 2. Recognition of single-molecular event

(PDMS) micro-fluid channel. Table 10.1 presents the classification of advanced biosensor materials and their applications.

10.3 APPLICATION OF BIOSENSORS

The recent developments in nanoscience and Nanotechnology have influenced enhancements and improvisations in biosensing technology, leading to development of sophisticated nanobiosensors. Nanobiosensors are broadly utilized in the domain of medical science to diagnose and monitor patient health. Nanobiosensors have some specific essential requirements, such as sensitivity, precision, stability and reproducibility for performing medical diagnosis and analysis of certain diseases [23, 24]. Nanobiosensors are utilized in various applications for medical diagnosis/analysis such as the detection of cancer or tumor biomarkers, detection of pathogenic viruses and bacteria, detection of allergic responses, detection of glucose and cholesterol levels and bio-imaging.

Early phase diagnosis is essential for the prevention of cancer, and involves detection of altered genes and proteins that are responsible for breakdown of the cellular pathways. The recent contrast agents and materials of nanobiosensors can help in prior and more precise initial investigation of cancer cells, together with continuous and periodic following of cancer patient therapy [25]. The sensors perform capturing of cancer cells or targeting of proteins using nanoscale tools, whereby the sensors get covered up by cancer antibodies or biorecognition ligands, after which an electrical/mechanical/optical signal is recognized [26]. Early detection of cancer in body liquids like serum and blood can also be done with the help of bio-conjugated particles. Superparamagnetic iron oxide nanoparticles (MNP) incorporated onto an antigen have been used to find the concentration of protein-tumor-markers using a sensitive identification methodology [27]. Nanobiosensors can detect nucleic acids, receptors, secretaries, biorecognition molecules and protein biomarkers. The most essential aspect is that the biosensor must be able to recognize the most appropriate biomarker which helps in molecular identification of particular antibodies and antigens.

Various infectious diseases, caused by viruses such as dengue, influenza, encephalitis and HIV, are on the rise and can spread through an enormous number of people in a small span of time [28–30]. Besides common laboratory diagnostic techniques, the use of biosensors and biochips have resulted in the introduction of enhanced modern diagnostic techniques that will soon become prominent due to low cost and simplicity in their procedure and functionality. HIV infections can now be identified by biosensors that use high-quality and sensitive diagnostic techniques based on electrochemistry. Nanofabrication techniques have also been improved to develop nano plasmonic biosensors [31]. The plasmon (optical) detection technique for quantifiable recognition of HIV-1 particles is established on a confined plasmon resonance mechanism. Such techniques can also be combined with analytical methods like Raman spectroscopy to detect viruses, along with their specific components, using enhanced and more accurate diagnostic parameters [32]. Such diagnostic systems are efficiently used in various applications, but further improvements are required to integrate sophisticated sensor arrays with nano- and microfluidic systems and nanoscale electronic components to develop effective diagnostic systems in the biomedical field [33, 34].

Biosensing technology is also used for identification of bacterial pathogens for food security tracking. Nanosensor systems use nanomaterials with biological-systems for increased response time and sensitivity [35, 36]. Nanomaterials like single-walled carbon nanotubes (SWCNTs) form the basic structure units for nanosensor-systems on account of their quality electrical, mechanical, structural and chemical characteristics. SWCNTs and immobilized antibodies have been included in a throwaway bio-nano junction sensor for recognition of *E. coli* K-12 [37, 38]. Graphene based nano-electronic biosensors are also used particularly for identifying gas-molecule-metal-ions and biomolecules like bacteria, glucose, proteins and DNA [39]. MOS image-based sensors have also emerged in the medical diagnostics field for detection of bacterial pathogens [40].

It has been observed that many consumers of food products suffer from food hypersensitivity and allergic reactions. Some common allergic reaction producing materials are proteins from milk and eggs, or nuts like peanuts among others. Nanobiosensors used for detection of these allergic substances in foodstuffs offer high responsiveness and sensitivity which is dependent on the number of analysts which are linked to the sensor's electrode [41]. Nanostructured biosensors with consistently accumulated gold-nanoparticles (GNPs) are used for sensing a minimum level of serum acquisition that is required for IgE (Immunoglobulin E) measurement in an allergic patient [42, 43].

It is cumbersome for diabetic patients to take frequent small blood samples in order to track and monitor the body's glucose levels. Medical nanorobotics can solve this problem by continuous tracking of the glucose level [44]. Nanocomposite membranes consisting of film-by-film assembly of carbon nanotubes (CNTs) including gold-nanoparticles (GNPs) are used for glucose biosensors [45]. Advanced nanomaterials or polymers can be combined with CNTs to develop advanced nanocomposites which are capable of offering enhanced facets and surface area for catalytic activities [46]. The CNTs are also combined with nanometals like gold, palladium and silver to increase the sensing capabilities of the glucose biosensor. Quantum dots (Qds) like CdS, CdSe, CdTe and ZnS have also been used in the development of GOx-based electrochemical and photo-electrochemical glucose biosensors, as QDs offer better electron transfer reactivity [47–49].

The essential part of the nerve cell and originator of numerous biomaterials like steroid hormones and bile acid are cholesterol and fatty acids [50]. These are vital parameters for a patient, and irregularities in the levels can cause serious ailments like high blood pressure, hyperthyroidism, coronary artery, anemia and so on. Hence, it becomes quite important to periodically monitor the cholesterol level of a patient. Cholesterol biosensors are made up of cholesterol oxidase (ChOx) which can be immobilized by applying nickel hexa-cyanoferrate nanoparticles (NiNPs) on histidine personalized CNT-based matrices [51]. Some cholesterol biosensors are also based on multi-walled carbon nanotubes (MWCNT) and improved carbon electrodes [52]. Such biosensors for cholesterol measurement have shown high sensitivity and quick response time, thus gaining a high level of acceptability.

Developments in nanotechnology and molecular level analysis have led to the usage of nanoparticles (NP) for modern disease diagnostics including bio-imaging. NPs such as gold nanoparticles, nanorods, Qds, manganese oxide and superparamagnetic iron oxide are being used in multimodal and multifunctional molecular imaging [53]. These NPs have features like surface plasmonic resonance, photoluminescence, paramagnetism and so on for appropriate molecular imaging [54]. Multifunctional nanoparticles are used for magnetic resonance imaging, various types of tomography, fluorescent imaging, ultrasound and photoacoustic imaging [53]. CNTs like MWNTs and SWNTs are also utilized in biomedical imaging. The usage of NP technology in biomedical imaging helps in early detection of a disease in its initial phase and, sometimes, even before the disease is about to develop [55].

10.4 CONCLUSION

This chapter demonstrates that the advancement in nanotechnology has improved the diagnosis and monitoring of health of a patient. Biosensors are widely used in medicines, clinical care and food processing, due to the character of trained molecules. Recent types of biosensors are briefly investigated in this chapter, and the use of these sensors in monitoring human health has been explained. Biosensors can be used to diagnose diseases by monitoring the blood glucose level, cholesterol level, and allergic level among others. Biosensors can be utilized to recognize micro-organisms such as viruses, bacteria and fungi. Advanced nanobiosensors have been utilized for recognition of pathogenic bacteria, viruses and cancer biomarkers. Nanoparticles are also used for molecular imaging to diagnose diseases.

REFERENCES

1. Adhikari B, Majumdar S, "Polymers in sensor applications", *Prog Polym Sci* 2004; 29: 699–766.
2. Scognamiglio V, "Nanotechnology in glucose monitoring: advances and challenges in the last 10 years", *Biosens Bioelectron* 2013; 47: 12–25.
3. Anker JN, Hall WP, Lyandres O, Shah NC, Zhao J, Van Duyne RP, "Biosensing with plasmonic nanosensors", *Nat Mater* 2008; 7: 442–453.
4. Sotiropoulou S, Gavalas V, Vamvakaki V, Chaniotakis NA, "Novel carbon materials in biosensor systems", *Biosens Bioelectron* 2002; 18: 211–5.
5. Mohankumar P, Ajayan J, Yasodharan R, Devendran P, Sambasivam R, "A review of micromachined sensors for automotive applications", *Measurement* 2019; 140: 305–322.
6. Ponmozhi J, Frias C, Marques T, Frazão O, "Smart sensors/actuators for biomedical applications", *Measurement* 2012; 45: 1675–1688.
7. Ronkainen NJ, Halsall HB, Heineman WR, "Electrochemical biosensors", *Chem Soc Rev* 2.
8. Chandrasekaran AR, Wady H, Subramanian HKK, "Nucleic acid nanostructures for chemical and biological sensing", *Small* 2016; 12: 2689–700.
9. Shacham-Diamand Y, Belkin S, Rishpon J, Elad T, Melamed S, Biran A, Yagur-Kroll S, Almog R, Daniel R, Ben-Yoav H, Rabner A, Vernick S, Elman N, Popovtzer R, "Optical and electrical interfacing technologies for living cell biochips", *Curr Pharm Biotechnol* 2010; 11: 376–83.
10. Soyer OS, Salathe M, Bonhoeffer S., "Signal transduction networks: topology, response and biochemical processes", *J Theor Biol* 2006; 238: 416–25.
11. Crew A, Lonsdale D, Byrd N, Pittson R, Hart JP., "A screen-printed, amperometric biosensor array incorporated into a novel automated system for the simultaneous determination of organophosphate pesticides", *Biosens Bioelectron* 2011; 26: 2847–51.
12. McNaught AD, Wilkinson A, *Compendium of Chemical Terminology*, IUPAC recommendations, 1997.
13. Lee SH, Sung JH, Park TH, "Nanomaterial-based biosensor as an emerging tool for biomedical applications", *Ann Biomed Eng* 2012; 40: 1384–1397.

14. Wise K, Weissman R, "Thin films of glass and their application to biomedical sensors", *Med Biological Eng* 1971; 9: 339–350.
15. Wang W, Lynch JP, "Application of guided wave methods to quantitatively assess healing in osseointegrated prostheses", *Struct Health Monit* 2018; 17: 1377–1392.
16. Jian M, Wang C, Wang Q, Wang H, Xia K, Yin Z, Zhang M, Liang X, Zhang Y, "Advanced carbon materials for flexible and wearable sensors", *Science China Materials* 2017; 60: 1026–1062.
17. Chen X, Park YJ, Kang M, Kang S-K, Koo J, Shinde SM, Shin J, Jeon S, Park G, Yan Y, "CVD-grown monolayer MoS2 in bioabsorbable electronics and bio-sensors", *Nat Commun* 2018; 9: 1–12.
18. Shin J, Yan Y, Bai W, Xue Y, Gamble P, Tian L, Kandela I, Haney CR, Spees W, Lee Y, "Bioresorbable pressure sensors protected with thermally grown silicon dioxide for the monitoring of chronic diseases and healing processes", *Nature Biomedical Engineering* 2019; 3: 37–46.
19. Carreiro S, Smelson D, Ranney M, Horvath KJ, Picard RW, Boudreaux ED, Hayes R, Boyer EW, "Real-time mobile detection of drug use with wearable biosensors: A pilot study", *J Med Toxicol* 2015; 11: 73–79.
20. Wang J, "Electrochemical glucose biosensors", *Chem Rev* 2008; 108: 814–825.
21. Liu S, Guo X, "Carbon nanomaterials field-effect-transistor-based biosensors", *NPG AsiaMaterials* 2012; 4: e23–e23.
22. Im H, Huang X-J, Gu B, Choi Y-K, "A dielectric-modulated field-effect transistor for biosensing", *Nat Nanotechnol* 2007; 2: 430.
23. Gdowski A, Ranjan AP, Mukerjee A, Vishwanatha JK, "Nanobiosensors: role in cancer detection and diagnosis", *Adv Exp Med Biol* 2014; 807: 33–58.
24. Singh RP, Oh BK, Choi JW, "Application of peptide nucleic acid towards development of nanobiosensor arrays", *Bioelectrochemistry* 2010; 79: 153–61.
25. Sanna V, Pala N, Sechi M, "Targeted therapy using Nanotechnology: focus on cancer", *Int J Nanomedicine* 2014; 9: 467–83.
26. Hessvik NP, Sandvig K, Llorente A, "Exosomal miRNAs as biomarkers for prostate cancer", *Front Genet* 2013; 4: 36.
27. Laurent S, Mahmoudi M. "Superparamagnetic iron oxide nanoparticles: promises for diagnosis and treatment of cancer", *Int J Mol Epidemiol Genet* 2011; 2: 367–90.
28. Kalthoff D, Globig A, Beer M, "(Highly pathogenic) avian influenza as a zoonotic agent", *Vet Microbiol* 2010; 140: 237–45.
29. Meng XJ, "Emerging and Re-emerging swine viruses", *Transbound Emerg Dis* 2012; 59: 85–102.
30. Karl S, Halder N, Kelso JK, Ritchie SA, Milne GJ, "A spatial simulation model for dengue virus infection in urban areas", *BMC Infect Dis* 2014; 14: 1–17.
31. Rifat AA, Ahmed R, Yetisen AK, Butt H, Sabouri A, Mahdiraji GA, Yun SH, Adikan FRM, "Photonic crystal fiber based plasmonic sensors", *Sens Actuators B* 2017; 243: 311–25.
32. Cao J, Sun T, Grattan KTV, "Gold nanorod-based localized surface plasmon resonance biosensors: a review", *Sens Actuators B* 2014; 195: 332–51.
33. Wilson AD, Baietto M, "Advances in electronic-nose technologies developed for biomedical applications", *Sensors* 2011; 11: 1105–76.
34. Wolfrum B, Kätelhön E, Yakushenko A, Krause KJ, Adly N, Hüske M, Rinklin P, "Nanoscale electrochemical sensor arrays: redox cycling amplification in dual electrode systems", *Acc Chem Res* 2016; 49: 2031–40.

35. Chen A, Chatterjee S, Nanomaterials based electrochemical sensors for biomedical applications", *Chem Soc Rev* 2013; 42: 5425.
36. Malhotra BD, Srivastava S, Ali MA, Singh C, "Nanomaterial-based biosensors for food toxin detection", *Appl Biochem Biotechnol* 2014; 174: 880–96.
37. Alpatova AL, Shan W, Babica P, Upham BL, Rogensues AR, Masten SJ, Drown E, Mohanty AK, Alocilja EC, Tarabara VV, "Single-walled carbon nanotubes dispersed in aqueous media via non-covalent functionalization: effect of dispersant on the stability, cytotoxicity, and epigenetic toxicity of nanotube suspensions", *Water Res* 2010; 44: 505–20.
38. Adhikari BR, Govindhan M, Chen A, "Carbon nanomaterials based electrochemical sensors/biosensors for the sensitive detection of pharmaceutical and biological compounds", *Sensors (Switzerland)* 2015; 15: 22490–508.
39. Varghese SS, Lonkar S, Singh KK, Swaminathan S, Abdala A, "Recent advances in graphene based gas sensors", *Sens Actuators B* 2015; 218: 160–83.
40. De Locht C, Van Den Broeck H, "Complementary metal-oxide-semiconductor (CMOS) image sensors for automotive applications" In: Daniel Durini (ed) *High Perform Silicon Imaging* Woodhead Publishing Series in Electronic and Optical Materials. 2014; 1: 235–49.
41. Kim J, Imani S, de Araujo WR, Warchall J, Valdés-Ramírez G, Paixaõ TRLC, Mercier PP, Wang J, "Wearable salivary uric acid mouthguard biosensor with integrated wireless electronics", *Biosens Bioelectron* 2015; 74: 1061–8.
42. Liu YF, Tsai JJ, Chin YT, Liao EC, Wu CC, Wang GJ, "Detection of allergies using a silver nanoparticle modified nanostructured biosensor", *Sens Actuators B* 2012; 171–172: 1095–100.
43. Peters RL, Gurrin LC, Dharmage SC, Koplin JJ, Allen KJ, "The natural history of IgEmediated food allergy: can skin prick tests and serum-specific IgE predict the resolution of food allergy?" *Int J Environ Res Public Health* 2013; 10: 5039–61.
44. Zhang W, Du Y, Wang ML, "Noninvasive glucose monitoring using saliva nanobiosensor", *Sens Biosens Res* 2015; 4: 23–9.
45. Zhu Z, Song W, Burugapalli K, Moussy F, Li YL, Zhong XH, "Nanoyarn carbon nanotube fiber based enzymatic glucose biosensor", *Nanotechnology* 2010; 21: 165501.
46. Tang H, Yan F, Lin P, Xu J, Chan HLW, "Highly sensitive glucose biosensors based on organic electrochemical transistors using platinum gate electrodes modified with enzyme and nanomaterials", *Adv Funct Mater* 2011; 21: 2264–72.
47. Amelia M, Lincheneau C, Silvi S, Credi A, "Electrochemical properties of CdSe and CdTe quantum dots", *Chem Soc Rev* 2012; 41: 5728.
48. Wang YF, Wang HY, Li ZS, Zhao J, Wang L, Chen QD, Wang WQ, Sun HB, "Electron extraction dynamics in CdSe and CdSe/CdS/ZnS quantum dots adsorbed with methyl viologen", *J Phys Chem C* 2014; 118: 17240–6.
49. Zhang J, Feng M, Tachikawa H, "Layer-by-layer fabrication and direct electrochemistry of glucose oxidase on single wall carbon nanotubes", *Biosens Bioelectron* 2007; 22: 3036–41.
50. Klaassen CD, Aleksunes LM, "Xenobiotic, bile acid, and cholesterol transporters", *Pharmacol Rev* 2014; 62: 1–96.
51. Gupta VK, Norouzi P, Ganjali H, Faridbod F, Ganjali MR, "Flow injection analysis of cholesterol using FFT admittance voltammetric biosensor based on MWCNT-ZnO nanoparticles", *Electrochim Acta* 2013; 100: 29–34.

52. Wang C, Tan X, Chen S, Yuan R, Hu F, Yuan D, Xiang Y, "Highly-sensitive cholesterol biosensor based on platinum-gold hybrid functionalized ZnO nanorods", *Talanta* 2012; 94: 263–70.
53. Padmanabhan P, Kumar A, Kumar S, Chaudhary RK, Gulyás B, "Nanoparticles in practice for molecular-imaging applications: an overview", *Acta Biomater* 2016; 41: 1–16.
54. Padmanabhan P, Kumar A, Kumar S, Chaudhary RK, Gulyás B, "Nanoparticles in practice for molecular-imaging applications: An overview", *Acta Biomater* 2016; 41: 1–16.
55. Veiseh O, Gunn JW, Zhang M, "Design and fabrication of magnetic nanoparticles for targeted drug delivery and imaging", *Adv Drug Deliv Rev* 2010; 62: 284–304.

Chapter 11

An Overview of Recent Progress in the Field of Wearable Glucose Sensors for Diabetes Diagnosis

Chandni Tiwari, Varun Mishra and Srishti

Graphic Era (deemed to be a University), Uttarakhand, India

CONTENTS

ABBREVIATIONS

CGM	Continuous glucose monitoring
CNT	Carbon nanotubes
FAD	Flavin adenine dinucleotide
ISF	Interstitial fluid
MOF	Metal organic framework
MWCNT	Multi-walled carbon nanotube
NAD	Nicotinamide adenine dinucleotide
PB	Phosphate buffer
WHO	World Health Organization

11.1 INTRODUCTION

Our modern human lifestyle has resulted in numerous diseases, and diabetes is one such illness which has affected many people. The normal blood glucose level in the fasting human body ranges from 3.9–6.1mmol/L [1].

DOI: 10.1201/9781003431138-11

An excess of glucose leads to various disease such as cardiovascular problems, blindness and retinal failures [2]. Apart from that, this ailment has been one of the major causes of death around the globe. Type1 and Type 2 diabetes result from decreased pancreatic β-cells, further creating shortage of insulin and target cell resistance, respectively [3]. Type 1 affects 5–10% and Type 2 affects 90–95% of total diabetic patients globally [4]. In a report published by the World Health Organization (WHO), diabetes is the seventh leading cause of human mortality [5]. Hence, maintenance of blood glucose within the physiological range is essential, along with its optimal management, and for this a blood monitoring system is required. Blood monitoring is widely categorized into two types: invasive and non-invasive.

Invasive methods are conventional and require blood samples drawn from a patient's body [6].These methods are painful and impose the risk of infections. Simultaneously, they also impose a limit on the number of tests done on patients. Non-invasive methods rely on other fluids extracted from the body and, hence, offer ease and comfort, along with an unlimited number of tests performed. Research efforts have been made since 1980 to develop a self-operatable glucose monitoring system [7]. The devices developed have been widely used by patients and utilize various enzyme-electrode strips. However, the methods of testing are invasive, as they require drawing of blood from a finger, and this results in limited frequency of testing. In the last few years, major improvements have been made in these devices to enhance performance such as speed, size, sensing mechanism, accuracy, production and ability to be "smart" devices [8]. These glucose sensors lack the ability to determine actual glucose level during sleep as it requires physical activity for accurate measurement. This need has resulted in the development and commercialization of non-invasive continuous glucose monitoring (CGM) systems.

The CGM system provides real-time detailed information of glucose levels and their rate of change for 24×7, along with alarm systems for hyper- and hypoglycemia, which is not the case in conventional systems [9]. These systems offer full information throughout the day regarding magnitude, frequency, direction and duration of glucose levels which leads to enhanced treatment of the disease. Such technology has been researched over the past few years which has resulted in few commercial CGM systems. These devices need to be implanted in the skin to measure the glucose level, through skin interstitial fluids, throughout the day [10]. Although these systems are minimally invasive, they are still less popular than invasive systems as they affect glycemic control. A completely non-invasive system, however, addresses all these problems and is an ideal system to control the disease before it impacts the human body severely. The last two decades have witnessed major efforts in development of various optical and electrochemical non-invasive glucose sensors. Although extensive research has been conducted in this field, a reliable and stable non-invasive CGM system is still required.

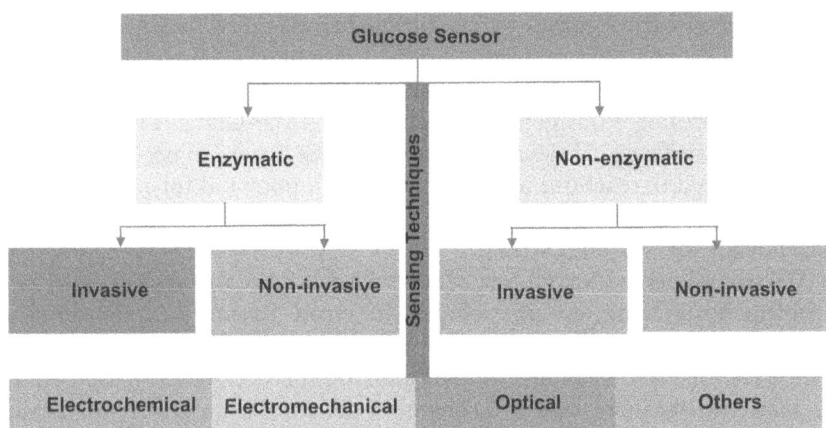

Figure 11.1 Schematic representation of various glucose sensors and their detection techniques.

Non-invasive techniques measure glucose levels from biofluids such as saliva, tears, interstitial skin fluid and sweat, rather than blood [2, 9]. The major challenges are the low concentration of glucose in biofluids in comparison to blood, and the techniques required to read this. The various detection techniques (utilizing the interaction of light with materials) include coherence, polarization, luminescence and scattering, to read the glucose level [11]. The device platform utilizes various wearable means such as watches, contact lens, and skin-patches. These detection techniques and the device platform offer a wide area for research [9]. The schematic of different glucose sensors and their sensing technique is shown in Figure 11.1.

The first section of this chapter is an introduction to electrochemical glucose sensors. Next, we discuss the materials utilized in these sensors along with their performance and their development in recent years. Later, we provide an overview of wearable glucose sensors, techniques of detection, limitations and prospects. Finally, the chapter is concluded with prospects in the field of wearable sensors.

11.2 EVOLUTION OF GLUCOSE SENSORS

Glucose sensors have evolved through time and can be classified in three generations. Enzymatic glucose sensors are one type, and they have been widely studied through the years. These glucose sensors use certain enzymes which are selective to glucose biomolecules. The most frequently used enzyme is glucose oxidase, which has high selectivity toward glucose molecules and can also work under variable pH and temperature in comparison to other counterparts [12]. Other major enzymes which have been used are glucose dehydrogenases which are further classified based on their co-factors. The co-factors pyrroloquinoline quinone (PQQ)-GDH and flavin adenine dinucleotide (FAD) tightly adhere to the enzymes. Whereas another co-factor, nicotinamide adenine dinucleotide (NAD)-GDH, is not bound to the enzyme surface [13]. These enzymes produce hydrogen peroxide (H_2O_2) during the redox reaction, which required high potential for measurement. Another concern about these first-generation glucose sensors was their dependency on oxygen [14, 15].

The second-generation glucose sensors tried to solve the oxygen deficiency problem by utilizing non-physiological electron acceptors to shuttle electrons. Various redox polymers, like poly(vinylimidazole) or poly(vinylpyridine), which are linked to osmium-complex electron relays covalently, are used to decrease the distance of the FAD center of the enzyme and the redox center of the polymer [14, 16]. This enables the sensors to have large current and fast response time. Other materials such as carbon nanotubes (CNT) and gold nanoparticles have been also used as an electrical connector between FAD center and electrode, owing to their comparable size [17].

The third-generation glucose sensors try to avoid the use of enzymes for sensing. Furthermore, they attempt to use materials which allow the direct transfer of electrons after sensing glucose to the electrode [18]. These are known as non-enzymatic glucose sensors. These glucose sensors avoid the complications used in the first two generations, and deliver ease of production [19]. However, selectivity is the major challenge faced by these sensors and this has been an open and active topic of research. Further, flexible and wearable glucose sensors, which have been also investigated over the years to allow a continuous monitoring of glucose, are also a part of this generation.

11.3 WEARABLE GLUCOSE SENSORS

In the last few years, new developments and technological advancements in wearable sensors have taken place in various fields such as environmental and biomedical. These wearable sensors use various liquids such as saliva, tears, sweat and interstitial fluid to measure glucose, rather than using blood. These sensors consist of an electrode to sense the glucose molecule along with a transducer to convert the reading into an electrical and measurable signal [20]. The sensors using sweat offer the availability of the fluid and its easy collection for facilitation of particular biomolecules for detection and amplification. There are various components such as cells, nucleic acids, receptors and enzymes which are used for detection in wearable biosensors. These are the building blocks for synthesis and characterization of biosensors, which use various sensing mechanisms such as calorimetric, optical and acoustic [6]. Despite major efforts to develop a fully non-invasive wearable glucose sensor, there are various issues which have occurred and need

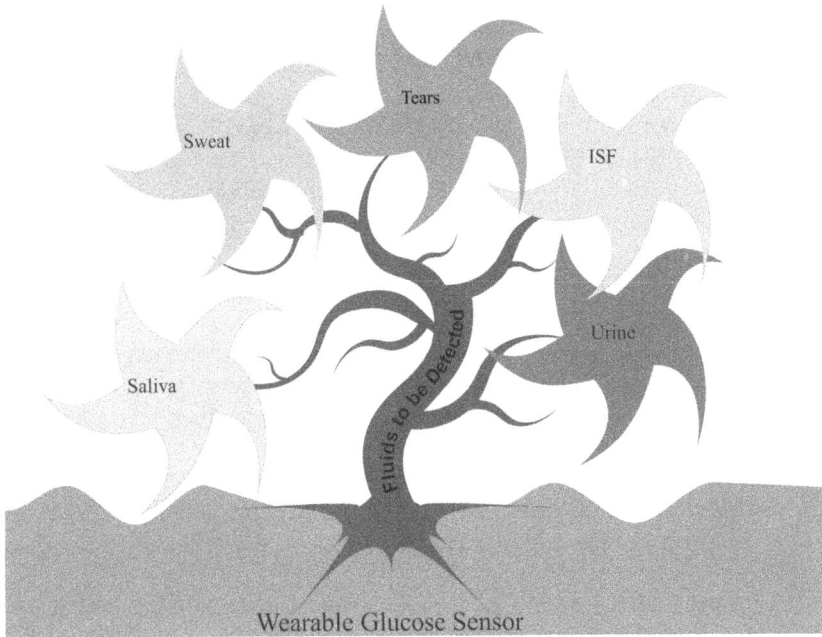

Figure 11.2 Different biofluids to be used in wearable glucose biosensor.

to be discussed. The bodily trait of external biofluids such as sweat, tears or saliva, presents problems as glucose sampling sites. These biofluids have a different composition for each person and are impacted by outer conditions such as humidity, moisture, air and physical activity [21]. Apart from that, the sweat has a different composition on different parts of the body, and the impact of residual sweat is also prominent in various bodily spots [22]. The sampling rate of sweat is variable and it requires electrical simulations. Similar issues exist with saliva flow, which does not have homogeneity in various spots of the mouth. It also has a different flow rate during day and night. Apart from that, saliva is affected by gum bleeding and, thus, suffers from glucose contamination. The availability of tears is limited which imposes restriction on continuous monitoring of glucose. Hence, due to these problems, mixed literature reports are available which relate these fluids to glucose concentration. The schematic of different fluids which is used in wearable sensors for sensing glucose is shown in Figure 11.2.

11.4 FLUIDS

Different body fluids which have been used to develop minimal invasive or non-invasive wearable glucose sensors are discussed in the following sections.

11.4.1 Sweat

Sweat is most easily accessible body fluid without inducing any discomfort in patients and it imposes low risk of contagion [23–25]. However, there are certain issues related to this fluid which we have discussed above [26]. To eradicate the above-mentioned problems, researchers have been trying to increase the sensitivity of sweat-based glucose sensors, so that they will require less volume of the fluid for glucose detection. Various substrates such as filter papers, patches, films and nanomaterials have been utilized by researchers to increase the sensitivity. Moreover, these materials have less thickness which ultimately reduces the size of the sensors and increases the ease of wearability. Filter papers are one of the most common choices for sweat-based sensors. Zhang et al. developed a low cost, self-powered and easily wearable sensor for glucose detection in sweat using Au/multiwalled carbon nanotube (MWCNT) and glucose dehydrogenase [27]. This sensor indicates a color change for changes in glucose concentration. This reduces the need for additional instruments, which leads to a less bulky and economical sensor. Further, a paper electrode was used to enhance the sensing of glucose.

Zheng et al. synthesized a carbon nanotube-based sweat-glucose sensor on filter paper [25]. Sweat collection is improved in this sensor by using a cloth-based sensor. This sensor was constructed using a low-cost screen-printed technique. The sensor showed excellent selectivity, stability and reproducibility, along with low production cost and could monitor for nine hours. Xiao et al. fabricated a sweat-glucose sensor based on cotton thread and filter paper [28]. The filter paper was functionalized by enzymes and reagents and high sensing performance was achieved. The capillary performance of cotton thread was enhanced with oxygen plasma prior to sensing.

Veeralingam et al. fabricated a RuS_2 nanoparticle deposited on a polydimethylsiloxane (PDMS) film-based sensor using a spin-coating technique [28]. This sensor was able to monitor pH level and glucose in sweat continuously in real time. Further, it was integrated with artificial intelligence. The sensor showed high accuracy and response time with excellent stability and reusability at room temperature. Bhide et al. synthesized a nano-porous electrode-based glucose sensor using ZnO thin film [29]. This sensor used oxidase of glucose and alcohol to functionalize the ZnO thin film, hence, making the sensor enzymatic in nature. The sensor used impedance spectroscopy to see the change in impedance after being exposed to glucose in the sweat sample. The sensor was able to sense 50–100mg/dl and showed excellent calibration. Lee et al. designed a patch-based sweat-glucose sensor [30]. This sensor had a multilayer patch and showed remarkable sensitivity. The sensor used a porous structure enabling a large number of glucose-sensing sites. They used phase-change material coated on hyaluronic acid hydrogel microneedles with two different phase-change materials. Xuan et al. used nanosheets of reduced graphene oxide (rGO) with a thin gold and platinum nanoparticles coating as a working electrode to sense glucose in sweat [31]. The composite was further deposited on a flexible polymide electrode by a facile low-cost technique. Further, glucose oxidase was decorated on the electrode to attain high sensitivity and selectivity. This sensor showed fast response, high sensitivity, linearity and large detection range. Oh et al. developed a stretchable and skin interfaced sweat glucose sensor which utilized cobalt tungstate ($CoWO_4$) as an electrode [32]. The electrodes were synthesized by using vacuum filtration of 60nm thin gold nanosheet through a template of polycarbonate. The multilayer CNT was deposited on the patterned gold electrode by a positively and negatively charged CNT solution. This increased the area and, hence, the sensitivity. Furthermore, one electrode was coated with $CoWO_4$/CNT nanocomposite which acted as a glucose sensor and another electrode was coated with poly-aniline (PANI) electrodeposition which acted as the pH sensor. This entire sensor except the electrode was subjected to silbione casing. This non-enzymatic stretchable and wearable sensor showed no interference from other sweat components, such as uric acid (UA), ascorbic acid (AA), acetaminophen (AP) and urea. The device showed high sensitivity and selectivity towards glucose molecules. Further, the authors compared this sensor's data with standard calorimetric results by recording the result from a human during physical activity over a day. The results were comparable and, hence, showed the potential of this device to act as a reliable, wearable glucose sensor. The sensor being firmly bound to the skin makes it difficult to extract the sweat required for continuous glucose monitoring. This issue has been addressed by Karpova et al. who proposed glucose monitoring from undiluted sweat just after excretion [33]. They used a phosphate buffer (PB) immobilized with GO_x enzyme in nafion or alkoxysilane gel. The alkoxysilane provided better sensitivity for a glucose range of $1\mu M$–$1mM$. The sweat was extracted by simulation of a minpilocarpine-based sweat gland on a spot of skin for 15 minutes. The sensor measured the current response from the sweat for flow duration of 20–30 minutes.

Although, there are several research papers available on sweat-based glucose sensors, there are various challenges that exist and need to be addressed. Apart from sampling problems, the major issue that exists is contamination of the sweat sample by the skin. The mixing of old and new sweat can also lead to changes in the actual value of glucose present in the sweat at a particular time [31]. Moreover, a large change in the pH of sweat (4.5–7.0) along with analytes present in eccrine glands will affect the actual value of glucose present in sweat [22]. Hence, these issues need to be eradicated to achieve a point-of-care, non-invasive and wearable sweat-based glucose sensor.

11.4.2 Saliva

Saliva is another attractive biofluid which has been utilized in continuous glucose monitoring. Several reports have emphasized the higher glucose concentration present in saliva obtained from diabetic humans [34, 35]. Also, the saliva sample collection is simple and does not require any sample pre-treatment, hence, making it a better choice for glucose monitoring. However, many reports have mentioned the need of saliva dilution and filtration prior to sensing [36]. Needless to say, apart from the convenience of collecting samples easily, this fluid offers some restrictions as well. The main component of saliva is water which makes the presence of another biomarker low [37, 38]. Castro et al. synthesized a wearable glucose sensor using paper-based substrate and saliva as the sample [39]. The realized device had a 3D printer holder along with a mouthguard made from silicon and electrode. This electrode was made from a simple low-cost technique and used a mixture of 4-aminoantipyrine (AAP) and 3,5-dichloro-2-hydroxybenzenesulfonic acid (DHBS) as a chromogenic solution. The insulation between reagents and mouth is provided by a 3D printed holder which mitigates the possibility of health hazards offered by chemical reagents which are water-soluble. This sensor used the sample without any pre-treatment and hence offered a low-cost, point-of-care wearable glucose sensor.

The higher sensitivity of these saliva-based sensors is also achieved by a metal-organic framework (MOF), using a non-enzymatic electrolytic reaction, which showed higher sensitivity. Wei et al. developed a non-enzymatic saliva-based glucose sensor for continuous monitoring [40]. They used a cobalt-based MOF modified carbon cloth on paper substrate as a hybrid and portable sensor. The Co-MOF acts as an artificial nanozyme which shows higher selectivity and sensitivity toward glucose detection. It also offers a low-cost and simple fabrication technique making it more favorable than enzymatic, wearable glucose sensors. In addition, the flexibility of the Co-MOF/CC interface integrated on paper offers sufficient sensing sites along with a large specific area. This button-sensor which is portable offers a comparable accuracy to the commercially available glucose sensors.

Recently, a sensor known as "cavitas sensor" was introduced by Arakava et al. [23]. This is a non-invasive sensor which measures glucose in saliva present in the human oral cavity. This sensor is made from platinum and an Ag/AgCl electrode fitted on a mouthguard support which is connected to a wireless transmitter. This sensor used immobilized GOx which was trapped into a matrix of methacrylate and meth-acryloyl phosphorylcholine-based copolymer. The glucose present in saliva can be found using telemetric measurement with the help of this sensor. This sensor resulted in a sensitivity in span of 0.05–1mM when tested on artificial saliva in a phantom jaw. Another work is reported by Garcia-Carmona et al. [41]. where they developed a pacifier integrated wearable sensor using a GOx–PB electrode transducer for monitoring glucose in a baby's saliva. The technique is continuous and non-invasive. When the baby sucks the pacifier, the efficient saliva is pumped through the mouth movement into electrode chamber. This sensor was further tested on Type 1 diabetes patients and has shown comparable results to a conventional glucometer.

11.4.3 Tears

Human tears are excreted from the lachrymal gland and act as a protective film which covers the eye [42]. They are usually a combination of over 20 different components such as electrolytes, water, proteins and trace metals among others [43]. The major problem associated with tear-based glucose monitoring is the collection of tear samples and the compromise of tear samples by any eye irritation or simulation [44]. The consumed glucose requires a minimum ten minutes to go to equilibrium in the blood and there is a five minute lag time between the appearance of glucose in blood and in tears [45]. Myopia has become a global health problem and vision correction can be done using contact lenses. Hence, smart contact lenses that could collect tears to monitor the glucose level has been studied recently by the research fraternity.

Ruan et al. have fabricated gelated, colloidal, crystal-based contact lenses for continuous glucose detection in tears [46]. The lens can sense glucose in the tears in the range of 0–50mM. The lens can emit wavelengths in the visible range of 567–468nm by sensing the change in glucose concentration. The color emitted is from reddish yellow to blue. This next-generation sensor has shown a small limit of detection (0.05mM) and the device is biocompatible, portable and induces no discomfort for the patients.

Guo et al. reported a MoS_2 transistor-based smart contact lens which is multifunctional [47]. They have used a PDMS lens substrate, on which MoS_2 nanosheets have been deposited which sense the glucose concentration in the tears. Apart from that, they used a photodetector, which sends optical information which is used to debug any corneal diseases. This mesh structure which is serpentine was directly integrated with the contact lens to improve sensitivity without affecting the vision of the patients. This lens showed great biocompatibility and could be used as a next-generation, wearable, smart glucose sensor for healthcare applications.

Another polymer-based lens is fabricated by Keum et al. and has shown an outstanding match with biomolecules [48]. This device is an integration of super thin soft circuits along with a microcontroller, data transmission and wireless supply system for sensing glucose in tears. The glucose concentration measured from this lens was further verified by glucose present in blood samples. This lens was also designed for drug delivery for diabetic retinopathy therapy. This device could be an asset to the healthcare industry in diabetes detection and to provide therapy.

An amperometric glucose sensor was introduced by Parviz's research group using a polymer substrate and microstructure deposition on the top of it [49]. The titania film deposited by a sol-gel method was subjected to immobilization of GOx which was further coated with nafion. The enzyme offers a high selectivity for glucose molecules, and nafion offers prevention of interference. The same group have extended this work by integrating the lens with a transmission system which is wireless to allow the real-time monitoring of glucose from tears. They have used an antenna in the form of loop for power supply and transfer of data with an electronic interface to read data. This device can be supplied with power from 15cm through wireless RF system. The data transmission was realized by a quite low power (3mW). This glucose sensor was tested continuously on a PDMS eye model which mimics the human eye and has shown a linear current response for the entire glucose detection range (0.1–0.6mM).

Sempionatto et al. demonstrated a glucose and vitamin marker-based eyewear for continuous and real-time monitoring [45]. The nose bridge of the eyewear is subjected to the fluidic system which simulates the tear flow from eye. The collected tears go to the biocatalytic detector. The enzyme used was GOx, which converts glucose into gluconic acid and H_2O_2 is released as a by-product. This by-product further reduces at a PB transducer with Ag/AgCl$_2$ as reference electrode at 0.2V. This eyewear is able to sense the glucose outside the eye, hence, it should be able to overcome the drawbacks faced by wearable contact lenses such as user compliance and vision impairment [50]. The most prominent challenge faced by these sensors is power supply. The power supply used in the device must be soft to avoid causing discomfort to the users. Researchers have shown lacrimal glucose and ascorbate as energy producing biofuel cells however, more studies need to be conducted in this area [51, 52].

11.4.4 Interstitial Fluid

The body's liquid environment is maintained by interstitial fluid (ISF) which is present between cells of the body [50, 53, 54]. The glucose concentration in ISF is higher, hence, reading glucose concentration from this would offer higher sensitivity and accuracy. For this reason, this fluid is an attractive choice for a glucose monitoring device.

Nightingale et al. realized a wearable glucose monitoring sensor using ISF which could provide high accuracy, resolution, small size and continuous monitoring [55]. It could monitor lactate and glucose in real time on volunteers. A patch-like ISF-based glucose monitor developed by Chen et al. used a gold electrode integrated with a flexible and thin paper-based battery. Hyaluronic acid (HA) was inserted into the ISF transdermally, using an anode channel by paper battery to increase its collection. The osmotic pressure of ISF is increased by positively charged HA which disrupts the balance between filtration and reabsorption of the ISF and promotes the flow of blood glucose into the ISF. The cathode channel extracts the ISF glucose, further it is detected by amperometric techniques using GO$_x$ enzymes. This sensor has San dunes-like nanostructures on gold thin film deposited on PMMA/polyimide substrate along with a PB transducer layer. The results obtained by this device were validated against the blood samples of the volunteers and have shown good correlations. An array of small pixels which contains a platinum functionalized graphene electrode was developed by

Lipani et al. and is non-invasive glucose patch working on a transdermal technique [56]. In this device, the sampling of the ISF is initiated by electro-osmotic extraction on a small skin area along the follicular path of the skin through an array of pixels integrated on the substrate. This method has shown better extraction capability by creating a pathway of extraction of the ISF with low resistance. It has shown high accuracy and calibration is not required in this device. They demonstrated the in vivo glucose monitoring in healthy human beings for six hours.

However, it is difficult to collect the ISF using non-invasive techniques, hence, it opens a new field of research. One method is the application of microneedles which reduces the wound caused by normal needles. Liu et al. fabricated a microneedle using polymer, where poly(ethylene glycol) (PEG) and polydopamine (PDA) were coated using a simple technique [57]. The PEG is hydrophilic and has anti-adhesion properties which makes the microneedle have high adhesion toward glucose and high speed of ISF extraction. The device has shown reliable accuracy in comparison to commercially available glucometers.

11.4.5 Urine

Urine is another fluid in which content of glucose is high which can be utilized for non-invasive glucose detection. Zhang et al. fabricated a glucose sensor attached with a diaper to sense glucose present in urine. It was also integrated with a biofuel which can generate electricity and provide power to the system. A power storage unit was also attached to store the generated power and the amount of glucose was indicated by a light emitted diode which shows different color corresponding to different concentration.

11.5 CONCLUSION

Wearable glucose sensors have become a prominent topic of research in recent years for continuous monitoring of diabetes. This chapter focused on the evolution of glucose sensors and the different fluids which are used to detect glucose for wearable sensors. The fluids of attention are sweat, saliva, tears, ISF and urine. Most of the research for wearable glucose sensors has focused on sweat, which is easy to collect and offers no discomfort. Tear-based glucose detection is also gaining attention and has led to synthesis of soft contact lenses to measure glucose. These lenses offer little discomfort and are useful for patients with myopia. The glucose sensor based on saliva needs more attention as it offers some challenges. The content of glucose in saliva is less and it is also affected by other factors. Further, it also needs filtration and dilution before testing. The wearable sensor based on ISF and urine also needs to be investigated further. These fluids are not available continuously and are in an initial stage of study.

The future prospects of these devices are bright, as developments in sensing material, transmission techniques and power supply are expected, which will lead to a small, accurate, and self-powered version of wearable glucose sensors. Further, these devices will replace the traditional glucose sensing instruments and users will have choice of the type of fluid which they want to be checked. The data can be monitored continuously and at home without any clinical expert and they can get the right treatment in good time.

REFERENCES

1. Coster, S., M. C. Gulliford, P. T. Seed, J. K. Powrie, and R. Swaminathan. 2000. "Monitoring Blood Glucose Control in Diabetes Mellitus: A Systematic Review." *Health Technology Assessment* 4 (12). https://doi.org/10.3310/hta4120

2. Peng, Zhiqing, Xiangyu Xie, Qilong Tan, Hu Kang, Ji Cui, Xia Zhang, Wang Li, and Guoying Feng. 2022. "Blood Glucose Sensors and Recent Advances: A Review." *Journal of Innovative Optical Health Sciences* 15 (02). https://doi.org/10.1142/S1793545822300038

3. Xiao, Gang, Jing He, Xiaodie Chen, Yan Qiao, Feng Wang, Qingyou Xia, Ling Yu, and Zhisong Lu. 2019a. "A Wearable, Cotton Thread/Paper-Based Microfluidic Device Coupled with Smartphone for Sweat Glucose Sensing." *Cellulose* 26 (7): 4553–62. https://doi.org/10.1007/s10570-019-02396-y

4. American Diabetes Association. 2014. "Diagnosis and Classification of Diabetes Mellitus." *Diabetes Care* 37 (Supplement_1): S81–90. https://doi.org/10.2337/dc14-S081

5. Adeel, Muhammad, Md. Mahbubur Rahman, Isabella Caligiuri, Vincenzo Canzonieri, Flavio Rizzolio, and Salvatore Daniele. 2020. "Recent Advances of Electrochemical and Optical Enzyme-Free Glucose Sensors Operating at Physiological Conditions." *Biosensors and Bioelectronics* 165 (October): 112331. https://doi.org/10.1016/j.bios.2020.112331

6. Zafar, Hima, Asma Channa, Varun Jeoti, and Goran M. Stojanović. 2022. "Comprehensive Review on Wearable Sweat-Glucose Sensors for Continuous Glucose Monitoring." *Sensors* 22 (2): 638. https://doi.org/10.3390/s22020638

7. Newman, Jeffrey D., and Anthony P.F. Turner. 2005. "Home Blood Glucose Biosensors: A Commercial Perspective." *Biosensors and Bioelectronics* 20 (12): 2435–53. https://doi.org/10.1016/j.bios.2004.11.012

8. Zhang, Sheng, Junyan Zeng, Chunge Wang, Luying Feng, Zening Song, Wenjie Zhao, Qianqian Wang, and Chen Liu. 2021. "The Application of Wearable Glucose Sensors in Point-of-Care Testing." *Frontiers in Bioengineering and Biotechnology* 9 (December). https://doi.org/10.3389/fbioe.2021.774210

9. Kim, Jayoung, Alan S. Campbell, and Joseph Wang. 2018. "Wearable Non-Invasive Epidermal Glucose Sensors: A Review." *Talanta* 177 (January): 163–70. https://doi.org/10.1016/j.talanta.2017.08.077

10. McGarraugh, Geoffrey. 2009. "The Chemistry of Commercial Continuous Glucose Monitors." *Diabetes Technology & Therapeutics* 11 (S1): S-17–S-24. https://doi.org/10.1089/dia.2008.0133

11. Rachim, Vega Pradana, and Wan-Young Chung. 2019. "Wearable-Band Type Visible-near Infrared Optical Biosensor for Non-Invasive Blood Glucose Monitoring." *Sensors and Actuators B: Chemical* 286 (May): 173–80. https://doi.org/10.1016/j.snb.2019.01.121

12. Heller, Adam, and Ben Feldman. 2008. "Electrochemical Glucose Sensors and Their Applications in Diabetes Management." *Chemical Reviews* 108 (7): 2482–2505. https://doi.org/10.1021/cr068069y

13. Teymourian, Hazhir, Abbas Barfidokht, and Joseph Wang. 2020. "Electrochemical Glucose Sensors in Diabetes Management: An Updated Review (2010–2020)." *Chemical Society Reviews* 49 (21): 7671–7709. https://doi.org/10.1039/D0CS00304B

14. Zhu, Zhigang, Luis Garcia-Gancedo, Andrew J. Flewitt, Huaqing Xie, Francis Moussy, and William I. Milne. 2012. "A Critical Review of Glucose Biosensors Based on Carbon Nanomaterials: Carbon Nanotubes and Graphene." *Sensors* 12 (5): 5996–6022. https://doi.org/10.3390/s120505996

15. Wang, Joseph. 2008. "Electrochemical Glucose Biosensors." *Chemical Reviews* 108 (2): 814–25. https://doi.org/10.1021/cr068123a

16. Pishko, Michael V., Ioanis Katakis, Sten-Eric Lindquist, Ling Ye, Brian A. Gregg, and Adam Heller. 1990. "Direct Electrical Communication between Graphite Electrodes and Surface Adsorbed Glucose Oxidase/Redox Polymer Complexes." *Angewandte Chemie International Edition in English* 29 (1): 82–84. https://doi.org/10.1002/anie.199000821

17. Patolsky, Fernando, Yossi Weizmann, and Itamar Willner. 2004. "Long-Range Electrical Contacting of Redox Enzymes by SWCNT Connectors." *Angewandte Chemie International Edition* 43 (16): 2113–17. https://doi.org/10.1002/anie.200353275

18. Hwang, Dae-Woong, Saram Lee, Minjee Seo, and Taek Dong Chung. 2018. "Recent Advances in Electrochemical Non-Enzymatic Glucose Sensors – A Review." *Analytica Chimica Acta* 1033 (November): 1–34. https://doi.org/10.1016/j.aca.2018.05.051

19. Tian, Kun, Megan Prestgard, and Ashutosh Tiwari. 2014. "A Review of Recent Advances in Nonenzymatic Glucose Sensors." *Materials Science and Engineering: C* 41 (August): 100–118. https://doi.org/10.1016/j.msec.2014.04.013

20. D'Orazio, Paul. 2003. "Biosensors in Clinical Chemistry." *Clinica Chimica Acta* 334 (1–2): 41–69. https://doi.org/10.1016/S0009-8981(03)00241-9.

21. Waltz, Emily. 2019. "Sweet Sensation." *Nature Biotechnology* 37 (4): 340–44. https://doi.org/10.1038/s41587-019-0086-2

22. Heikenfeld, Jason. 2016. "Non-Invasive Analyte Access and Sensing through Eccrine Sweat: Challenges and Outlook circa 2016." *Electroanalysis* 28 (6): 1242–49. https://doi.org/10.1002/elan.201600018

23. Arakawa, Takahiro, Yusuke Kuroki, Hiroki Nitta, Prem Chouhan, Koji Toma, Shin-ichi Sawada, Shuhei Takeuchi, et al. 2016. "Mouthguard Biosensor with Telemetry System for Monitoring of Saliva Glucose: A Novel Cavitas Sensor." *Biosensors and Bioelectronics* 84 (October): 106–11. https://doi.org/10.1016/j.bios.2015.12.014

24. Yu, Lan, Zhen Yang, and Ming An. 2019. "Lab on the Eye: A Review of Tear-Based Wearable Devices for Medical Use and Health Management." *BioScience Trends* 13 (4): 308–13. https://doi.org/10.5582/bst.2019.01178

25. Zheng, Lin, Yuan Liu, and Chunsun Zhang. 2021. "A Sample-to-Answer, Wearable Cloth-Based Electrochemical Sensor (WCECS) for Point-of-Care Detection of Glucose in Sweat." *Sensors and Actuators B: Chemical* 343 (September): 130131. https://doi.org/10.1016/j.snb.2021.130131

26. Sonner, Z., E. Wilder, J. Heikenfeld, G. Kasting, F. Beyette, D. Swaile, F. Sherman, et al. 2015. "The Microfluidics of the Eccrine Sweat Gland, Including Biomarker Partitioning, Transport, and Biosensing Implications." *Biomicrofluidics* 9 (3): 031301. https://doi.org/10.1063/1.4921039

27. Zhang, Xiaowei, Yin Jing, Qingfeng Zhai, You Yu, Huanhuan Xing, Jing Li, and Erkang Wang. 2018. "Point-of-Care Diagnoses: Flexible Patterning Technique for Self-Powered Wearable Sensors." *Analytical Chemistry* 90 (20): 11780–84. https://doi.org/10.1021/acs.analchem.8b02838

28. Xiao, Jingyu, Yang Liu, Lei Su, Dan Zhao, Liang Zhao, and Xueji Zhang. 2019b. "Microfluidic Chip-Based Wearable Colorimetric Sensor for Simple and Facile Detection of Sweat Glucose." *Analytical Chemistry* 91 (23): 14803–7. https://doi.org/10.1021/acs.analchem.9b03110

29. Bhide, Ashlesha, Sriram Muthukumar, and Shalini Prasad. 2018. "CLASP (Continuous Lifestyle Awareness through Sweat Platform): A Novel Sensor for Simultaneous Detection of Alcohol and Glucose from Passive Perspired Sweat." *Biosensors and Bioelectronics* 117 (October): 537–45. https://doi.org/10.1016/j.bios.2018.06.065

30. Lee, Hyunjae, Changyeong Song, Yong Seok Hong, Min Sung Kim, Hye Rim Cho, Taegyu Kang, Kwangsoo Shin, Seung Hong Choi, Taeghwan Hyeon, and Dae-Hyeong Kim. 2017. "Wearable/Disposable Sweat-Based Glucose Monitoring Device with Multistage Transdermal Drug Delivery Module." *Science Advances* 3 (3). https://doi.org/10.1126/sciadv.1601314

31. Xuan, Xing, Hyo S. Yoon, and Jae Y. Park. 2018. "A Wearable Electrochemical Glucose Sensor Based on Simple and Low-Cost Fabrication Supported Micro-Patterned Reduced Graphene Oxide Nanocomposite Electrode on Flexible Substrate." *Biosensors and Bioelectronics* 109 (June): 75–82. https://doi.org/10.1016/j.bios.2018.02.054

32. Oh, Seung Yun, Soo Yeong Hong, Yu Ra Jeong, Junyeong Yun, Heun Park, Sang Woo Jin, Geumbee Lee, et al. 2018. "Skin-Attachable, Stretchable Electrochemical Sweat Sensor for Glucose and PH Detection." *ACS Applied Materials & Interfaces* 10 (16): 13729–40. https://doi.org/10.1021/acsami.8b03342

33. Karpova, Elena V., Elizaveta V. Shcherbacheva, Andrei A. Galushin, Darya V. Vokhmyanina, Elena E. Karyakina, and Arkady A. Karyakin. 2019. "Noninvasive Diabetes Monitoring through Continuous Analysis of Sweat Using Flow-Through Glucose Biosensor." *Analytical Chemistry* 91 (6): 3778–83. https://doi.org/10.1021/acs.analchem.8b05928

34. Liu, Chengcheng, Yongjie Sheng, Yanhong Sun, Junkui Feng, Shijin Wang, Jin Zhang, Jiacui Xu, and Dazhi Jiang. 2015. "A Glucose Oxidase-Coupled DNAzyme Sensor for Glucose Detection in Tears and Saliva." *Biosensors and Bioelectronics* 70 (August): 455–61. https://doi.org/10.1016/j.bios.2015.03.070

35. Zhang, Wenjun, Yunqing Du, and Ming L. Wang. 2015. "Noninvasive Glucose Monitoring Using Saliva Nano-Biosensor." *Sensing and Bio-Sensing Research* 4 (June): 23–29. https://doi.org/10.1016/j.sbsr.2015.02.002

36. Ji, Suk, and Youngnim Choi. 2015. "Point-of-Care Diagnosis of Periodontitis Using Saliva: Technically Feasible but Still a Challenge." *Frontiers in Cellular and Infection Microbiology* 5 (September). https://doi.org/10.3389/fcimb.2015.00065

37. Czumbel, László Márk, Szabolcs Kiss, Nelli Farkas, Iván Mandel, Anita Hegyi, Ákos Nagy, Zsolt Lohinai, et al. 2020. "Saliva as a Candidate for COVID-19 Diagnostic Testing: A Meta-Analysis." *Frontiers in Medicine* 7 (August). https://doi.org/10.3389/fmed.2020.00465

38. Chiappin, Silvia, Giorgia Antonelli, Rosalba Gatti, and Elio F. De Palo. 2007. "Saliva Specimen: A New Laboratory Tool for Diagnostic and Basic Investigation." *Clinica Chimica Acta* 383 (1–2): 30–40. https://doi.org/10.1016/j.cca.2007.04.011

39. Castro, Lucas F. de, Soraia V. de Freitas, Lucas C. Duarte, João Antônio C. de Souza, Thiago R. L. C. Paixão, and Wendell K. T. Coltro. 2019. "Salivary Diagnostics on Paper Microfluidic Devices and Their Use as Wearable Sensors for Glucose Monitoring." *Analytical and Bioanalytical Chemistry* 411 (19): 4919–28. https://doi.org/10.1007/s00216-019-01788-0

40. Wei, Xiaofeng, Jialei Guo, Huiting Lian, Xiangying Sun, and Bin Liu. 2021. "Cobalt Metal-Organic Framework Modified Carbon Cloth/Paper Hybrid Electrochemical Button-Sensor for Nonenzymatic Glucose Diagnostics." *Sensors and Actuators B: Chemical* 329 (February): 129205. https://doi.org/10.1016/j.snb.2020.129205

41. García-Carmona, Laura, Aida Martín, Juliane R. Sempionatto, Jose R. Moreto, María Cristina González, Joseph Wang, and Alberto Escarpa. 2019. "Pacifier Biosensor: Toward Noninvasive Saliva Biomarker Monitoring." *Analytical Chemistry* 91 (21): 13883–91. https://doi.org/10.1021/acs.analchem.9b03379

42. Kim, Jayoung, Alan S. Campbell, Berta Esteban-Fernández de Ávila, and Joseph Wang. 2019. "Wearable Biosensors for Healthcare Monitoring." *Nature Biotechnology* 37 (4): 389–406. https://doi.org/10.1038/s41587-019-0045-y

43. Ohashi, Yoshiki, Murat Dogru, and Kazuo Tsubota. 2006. "Laboratory Findings in Tear Fluid Analysis." *Clinica Chimica Acta* 369 (1): 17–28. https://doi.org/10.1016/j.cca.2005.12.035

44. Farandos, Nicholas M., Ali K. Yetisen, Michael J. Monteiro, Christopher R. Lowe, and Seok Hyun Yun. 2015. "Contact Lens Sensors in Ocular Diagnostics." *Advanced Healthcare Materials* 4 (6): 792–810. https://doi.org/10.1002/adhm.201400504

45. Sempionatto, Juliane R., Laís Canniatti Brazaca, Laura García-Carmona, Gulcin Bolat, Alan S. Campbell, Aida Martin, Guangda Tang, et al. 2019. "Eyeglasses-Based Tear Biosensing System: Non-Invasive Detection of Alcohol, Vitamins and Glucose." *Biosensors and Bioelectronics* 137 (July): 161–70. https://doi.org/10.1016/j.bios.2019.04.058

46. Ruan, Jia-Li, Cheng Chen, Jian-Hua Shen, Xue-Ling Zhao, Shao-Hong Qian, and Zhi-Gang Zhu. 2017. "A Gelated Colloidal Crystal Attached Lens for Noninvasive Continuous Monitoring of Tear Glucose." *Polymers* 9 (12): 125. https://doi.org/10.3390/polym9040125

47. Guo, Shiqi, Kaijin Wu, Chengpan Li, Hao Wang, Zheng Sun, Dawei Xi, Sheng Zhang, et al. 2021. "Integrated Contact Lens Sensor System Based on Multifunctional Ultrathin MoS2 Transistors." *Matter* 4 (3): 969–85. https://doi.org/10.1016/j.matt.2020.12.002

48. Keum, Do Hee, Su-Kyoung Kim, Jahyun Koo, Geon-Hui Lee, Cheonhoo Jeon, Jee Won Mok, Beom Ho Mun, et al. 2020. "Wireless Smart Contact Lens for Diabetic Diagnosis and Therapy." *Science Advances* 6 (17). https://doi.org/10.1126/sciadv.aba3252

49. Yao, Huanfen, Angela J. Shum, Melissa Cowan, Ilkka Lähdesmäki, and Babak A. Parviz. 2011. "A Contact Lens with Embedded Sensor for Monitoring Tear Glucose Level." *Biosensors and Bioelectronics* 26 (7): 3290–96. https://doi.org/10.1016/j.bios.2010.12.042

50. Bandodkar, Amay J., and Joseph Wang. 2014. "Non-Invasive Wearable Electrochemical Sensors: A Review." *Trends in Biotechnology* 32 (7): 363–71. https://doi.org/10.1016/j.tibtech.2014.04.005

51. Falk, Magnus, Viktor Andoralov, Zoltan Blum, Javier Sotres, Dmitry B. Suyatin, Tautgirdas Ruzgas, Thomas Arnebrant, and Sergey Shleev. 2012. "Biofuel Cell as a Power Source for Electronic Contact Lenses." *Biosensors and Bioelectronics* 37 (1): 38–45. https://doi.org/10.1016/j.bios.2012.04.030

52. Falk, Magnus, Viktor Andoralov, Maria Silow, Miguel D. Toscano, and Sergey Shleev. 2013. "Miniature Biofuel Cell as a Potential Power Source for Glucose-Sensing Contact Lenses." *Analytical Chemistry* 85 (13): 6342–48. https://doi.org/10.1021/ac4006793

53. Potts, Russell O., Janet A. Tamada, and Michael J. Tierney. 2002. "Glucose Monitoring by Reverse Iontophoresis." *Diabetes/Metabolism Research and Reviews* 18 (S1): S49–53. https://doi.org/10.1002/dmrr.210

54. Lee, Hyunjae, Yongseok Joseph Hong, Seungmin Baik, Taeghwan Hyeon, and Dae-Hyeong Kim. 2018. "Enzyme-Based Glucose Sensor: From Invasive to Wearable Device." *Advanced Healthcare Materials* 7 (8): 1701150. https://doi.org/10.1002/adhm.201701150

55. Nightingale, Adrian M., Chi Leng Leong, Rachel A. Burnish, Sammer-ul Hassan, Yu Zhang, Geraldine F. Clough, Martyn G. Boutelle, David Voegeli, and Xize Niu. 2019. "Monitoring Biomolecule Concentrations in Tissue Using a Wearable Droplet Microfluidic-Based Sensor." *Nature Communications* 10 (1): 2741. https://doi.org/10.1038/s41467-019-10401-y

56. Lipani, Luca, Bertrand G. R. Dupont, Floriant Doungmene, Frank Marken, Rex M. Tyrrell, Richard H. Guy, and Adelina Ilie. 2018. "Non-Invasive, Transdermal, Path-Selective and Specific Glucose Monitoring via a Graphene-Based Platform." *Nature Nanotechnology* 13 (6): 504–11. https://doi.org/10.1038/s41565-018-0112-4

57. Liu, Pei, Hongyao Du, Zhuoli Wu, Hua Wang, Juan Tao, Lianbin Zhang, and Jintao Zhu. 2021. "Hydrophilic and Anti-Adhesive Modification of Porous Polymer Microneedles for Rapid Dermal Interstitial Fluid Extraction." *Journal of Materials Chemistry B* 9 (27): 5476–83. https://doi.org/10.1039/D1TB00873K

Chapter 12

A Perspective View for Detection of COVID-19 Causative Virus (SARS-Cov-2) Using Dielectric Modulated Field Effect Transistors

Saurabh Kumar and R. K. Chauhan
Madan Mohan Malaviya University of Technology, Gorakhpur, India

Vimal Kumar Mishra
Jaypee Institute of Information Technology, Noida, Uttar Pradesh, India

CONTENTS

ABBREVIATIONS

CDC	Centers for disease control and prevention
CMOS	Complementary metal oxide semiconductor
CNTs	Carbon nanotubes
CoV	Coronavirus
COVID-19	Coronavirus disease 2019
FET	Field effect transistor
HE	Hemagglutinin esterase
MOSFET	Metal oxide semiconductor field effect transistor
rGO	Reduced graphene oxide
RNA	Ribonucleic acid
SARS	Severe acute respiratory syndrome
SARS-CoV-2	Severe acute respiratory syndrome coronavirus 2
SOI	Silicon on insulator

DOI: 10.1201/9781003431138-12

TFET   Tunnel field effect transistor
TMDC   Transition metal dichalcogenide
VT   Threshold voltage

12.1 INTRODUCTION

The World Health Organization declared COVID-19 as a pandemic on March 11, 2019, ten decades after the "Spanish flu" pandemic (1918–1920) [1]. The COVID-19 pandemic created a very unpleasant situation around the globe due to the lockdowns and restrictions necessary to save lives [2]. The SARS-CoV-2 virus, the cause of COVID-19, is a respiratory syndrome belonging to (RNA) virus, that is, a single-stranded positive-sense ribonucleic acid, and it is also a member of the coronaviridae family [3]. The Severe Acute Respiratory Syndrome Coronavirus-2 (SARS CoV-2) genome is approximately 75–80% similar to SARS-CoV, so this virus causes the COVID-19 disease [4]. It has a crown-like structure called a "corona" [5]. This virus enters the human body through the eye, nose, and mouth and then moves into lung tissue: from there, the virus spreads to the body [6]. Although this virus belongs to the β-CoV genera, the exact source of the virus is still unknown. Scientists have found that bats and rodents are suitable candidates to typically derive the virus's gene source [7]. To design various diagnostic techniques, structural understanding, immunological, microbiology and neuropathology, details of SARS CoV-2 are required [8]. The Centers for Disease Control and Prevention (CDC), which are governed by the United States of America (USA), displayed the virus image as shown in Figure 12.1 [9]. The shape of

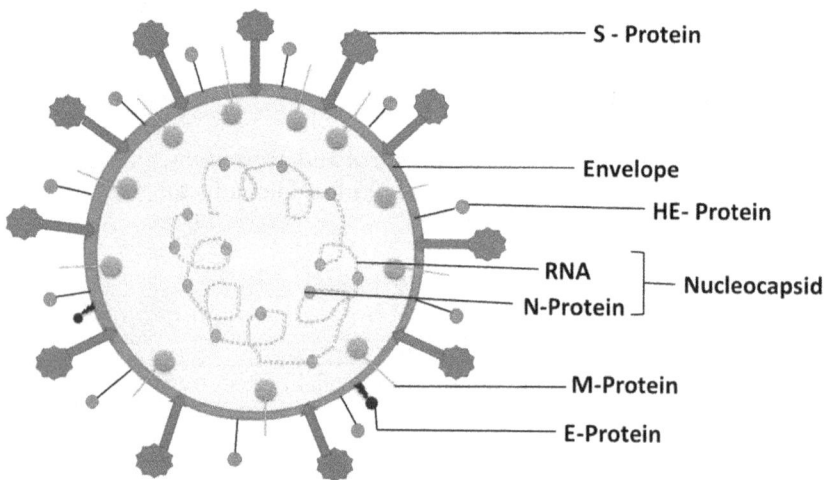

Figure 12.1 COVID-19 particle structure.

the virus basically consists of a thin membrane of a round shape in which spikes in the form of envelope protein are attached. For the detection of viruses, four structural proteins are important players. The first one is an envelope (E), the second one is a spike (S), the third one is nucleocapsid (N), and the fourth one is the matrix (M)[10–13]. Its genetic material, ribonucleic acid (RNA), is covered by nucleocapsid proteins (N-Protein). A hemagglutinin-esterase protein is also found in some coronaviruses (HE) [14].

12.2 AVAILABLE DETECTION METHODOLOGY

Developing an effective vaccine or treatment for such a virus is a challenge for many nations [15]. The approaches taken by world scientists to slow down the multiplying of this dangerous virus were through early identification and treatment [16]. At present, a common identification method used by doctors is nasopharyngeal, in which samples are taken from the nose and throat, and these samples are reported through real-time reverse transcription-polymerase chain reaction (RT-PCR) for three hours to identify SARS-CoV-2 in humans. Another approach is an IgG antibody through enzyme-linked immunosorbent assays (ELISA), also currently used to identify SARS-CoV-2 in humans. Moreover, as a further reduction of detection time of CoV-2, scientists propose one more approach, that is, mass spectrometry-based proteomics. The ELISA test basically looks at the corresponding antibodies present in the patient's blood serum instead of the actual virus.[17–18]. The most popular diagnostic technique is real-time RT-PCR, which uses a sample from an internal nasal swab to find E and N-protein genes, that is, RNA. This relies on complex devices and skilled operators [19]. The RT-PCR test is laborious and expensive and follows a time-consuming process. Researchers are enthusiastically advancing various diagnostic techniques to overcome problems and limitations related to present detection techniques to develop low-cost, reliable and rapid detection methods for the COVID-19 causative virus [20].

The COVID-19 virus is extremely contagious and spreads quickly throughout the world; COVID-19 spreads much more quickly than middle east respiratory syndrome (MERS) and SARS [21]. Additionally, reports of asymptomatic COVID-19 transmission have surfaced [22]. In the RT-PCR test, the data is taken in the real-time domain, which requires a minimum of three hours to complete a molecular diagnosis, including the synthesis of viral RNA [23]. The process of RNA preparation can also influence the accuracy of a diagnosis. Therefore, for the quick and precise diagnosis of COVID-19, highly sensitive immunological diagnostic techniques do not require sample preparation processes to find the different antigens of the virus.

12.3 FET-BASED BIOSENSORS

In the current scenario, a large amount of testing is required to detect the virus, so, as an alternative, biosensors might be potential candidates for detection as compared to the other current diagnostic methods to detect the COVID-19 causative virus, such as the RT-PCR and antigen and antibody tests. Biosensors may be viable since they provide great sensitivity and selectivity in detecting viral infections [24]. A typical biosensor is made up of three parts: the first one is a biological constituent, the second one is a transducer for translating the recognition process into a quantitative signal, and the third one is an electrical system for signal amplification and processing [25–27], as shown in Figure 12.2.

Furthermore, the transducers are categorized in terms of optical-based, electrochemical-based and FET-based. The optical and electrochemical-based biosensors are good options for real-time processing because they have excellent selectivity and low detection limits [28]. However, due to their quick screening and high sensitivity, the introduction of easier and potentially useful devices like FETs has gained increasing relevance. Some significant biosensing methods for detecting the COVID-19 causative virus and their characteristics are listed in Table 12.1.

Among these, FET-based biosensing devices provide numerous benefits, such as taking measurements instantly and with great sensitivity, even utilizing little or no analyte [35–36]. Thus, FET-based biosensors may be helpful for on-site detection, clinical diagnosis and point-of-care testing. The qualities of a FET-based biosensor that must be devised for effective application in pandemics are: High sensitivity, quick response time, mass manufacturability, long shelf-life, ease of use, and they must be cost-effective [37–40]; these qualities are depicted in Figure 12.3.

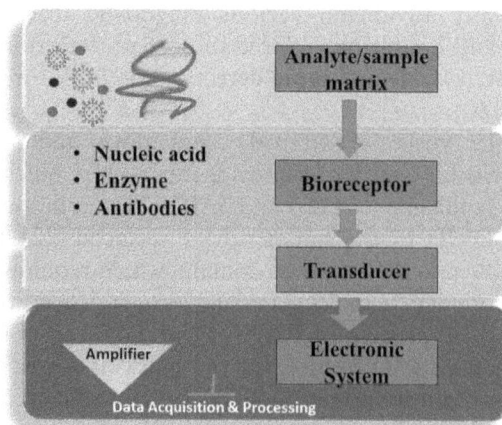

Figure 12.2 Illustration of typical biosensor component.

Table 12.1 Some important biosensing methods and their properties for detecting COVID-19 virus

Biosensor type	Properties
Plasmonic-based biosensors [29]	Biosensors which are based on plasmonic are basically label-free and impressively susceptible and can detect a variety of clinically relevant target analytes; for example, surface plasmonic resonance (SPR) biosensors can be applied to human serum samples without dilution to detect nucleocapsid, i.e., multifunctional protein antibodies.
FET-based biosensors [30–31]	Researchers have developed different FET-based biosensing devices such as MOSFET, FDSOI and TFET. These devices have several intriguing benefits, like instantly detecting minute amounts of the target analyte. These kinds of biosensors could be used for on-site diagnostics and clinical analyses.
Electrochemical-based biosensors [32–33]	Biosensors based on electrochemicals are used because of their simplicity, high sensitivity, low-cost and low fabrication complexity.
Optical biosensors [34]	Because they don't rely on any fluorescent or radiolabeling, optical biosensors are favored for their quick detection times, sensitivity and resilience. With the label-free approach, drug profiling false positives are reduced, and pricey labeling procedures are also avoided.

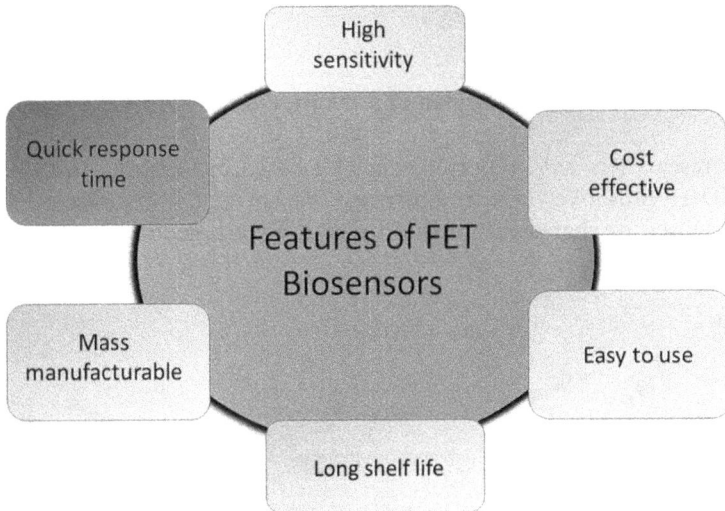

Figure 12.3 Features of an effective FET-based biosensor.

12.4 WORKING PRINCIPLES OF FET-BASED BIOSENSORS

Among a number of transducers in the category of label-free, FET-based biosensors are good options [41]. In contrast to microcantilever sensors, surface plasmon resonance, fluorescence devices and other available biosensor approaches, FET-based biosensors have important advantages such as rapid real-time detection, good portability, ultrasensitivity, inherent amplification, good scalability, lower power requirements, direct electrical readout and mass production at low costs. As a result, they have gained significantly more consideration in the current scenario. A major benefit of having established manufacturing processes like the metal oxide semiconductor (MOS) technology is that it facilitates the analogous sensing, miniaturization and assimilation of circuits and systems, which are crucial for the enlargement of practical real-time biosensing devices [42]. Target biomolecules carrying electrostatic charges or bioactivities that alter the device's electrostatic potential are generally preferred.

A MOS technology-based biosensor consists of three electrodes: gate, drain, and source. With the help of gate oxide and gate terminal, the biological identification facet intercepts the target analyte/biomolecules in between the drain and source, and detects the presence of the virus in terms of electrical and concentration phenomena. Finally, the biosensors directly convert the biological molecular data into an experimental signal. The signal which is obtained is amplified and processed for further application. An illustration of COVID-19 causative virus detection by an FET-based biosensor is shown in Figure 12.4.

12.5 RECENT DEVELOPMENTS IN FET-BASED BIOSENSORS

Many researchers have reported that FET-based biosensors can detect the COVID-19 causative virus. Among many, Parvin et al. [43] proposed a FET-based biosensor that uses transition metal dichalcogenide (TMDC) WSe2

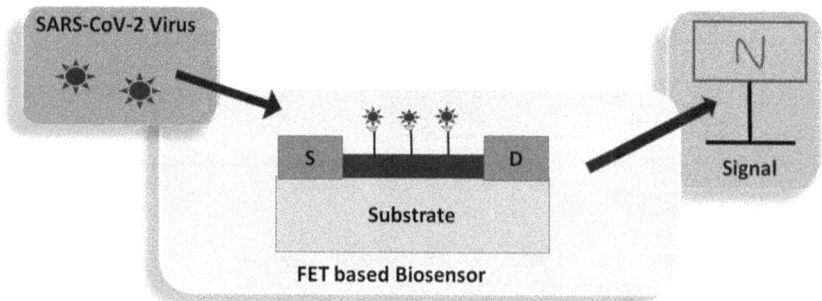

Figure 12.4 Detection of SARS-CoV-2 by FET-based biosensor.

for a sensitive and fast response while detecting the COVID-19 virus [43]. The findings of Parvin show that 2D-FETs based on TMDCs can be used to find the high sensitivity and better selectivity of biosensors for the rapid finding of infectious illnesses [43]. Mazin et al. (2022) proposed a CNT-FET electrochemical sensor for COVID-19 S1 antigen detection. The MOS-based biosensor showed better selectivity, high sensitivity, and fast response time, which could be a useful platform for quickly detecting COVID-19 S1 antigen in patients' nasopharyngeal saliva [44]. Vamsi et al. [45] worked to detect the COVID-19 causative virus using a reduced graphene oxide FET (rGO FET). They conclude that GFET is a powerful tool for swiftly screening viral proteins, tiny biomolecules and other biomarkers. The reported biosensors are particularly well-suited for future biomedical applications and can be effectively used to diagnose virus infection and lab-on-chip platforms [45]. From their work, it can be concluded that the FET-based biosensor can be used to detect the COVID-19 causative virus.

12.6 DIELECTRIC MODULATED FET (DMFET)-BASED BIOSENSORS

The possibility of incorporating bio-detection capabilities into present semiconductor technology is encouraged by the electrically operated gate of a DMFET, which controls the movement of charge across a semiconducting channel. Biosensors using DMFETs may sense surface changes from their surroundings and offer the best sensing conditions for ultrasensitive and low-noise detection. This makes applications involving sensitive immunological diagnosis using DMFET technology particularly appealing.

In several proposed FET biosensors, the gate or the channel is affected by the interaction of biomolecules [46–47]. In a DMFET device, when a voltage more than the threshold voltage (VT) is applied to the gate terminal, an electric current starts to flow from the source to the drain terminals. The threshold voltage is controlled by the gate capacitance; hence, we can modulate the threshold voltage of a DMFET by varying the dielectric constant of the gate oxide through the gate terminal [48]. Furthermore, with the introduction of biomolecules into the nanogap region, the gate capacitance increases as compared to the air gap capacitance, which shifts the threshold shifts of the device toward the negative direction. Therefore, it is possible to identify the various biomolecules present in the virus by keeping an eye on the threshold voltage change [49]. Rahul et al. (2021) presented analytical modeling of a DM double gate FET (DM-DGFET). As they demonstrated, the more the vertical silicon oxide (SiO_2) layers shift toward the source region, the better the gate controlling and, as a result, the higher the biosensor's sensitivity. The nanogap structure of an FET-based biosensor should be adjusted and improved, as per the size of the coronavirus, for an efficient way of detection [50]. Shivendra et al. (2020) proposed a structure that is essentially an enlarged version of a real device with work function engineering (plasma generation) and electrical doping modifications. According to the author, this device can be used for the competent detection of the SARS CoV-2 virus [51].

The complementary metal oxide semiconductor (CMOS) FET-based biosensor may be the best contender from all of the current diagnostic methods since it offers several advantages. One example is an instantaneous measurement with high sensitivity, even for extremely small amounts of analytes. SOI (Silicon on Insulator) offers improved channel control, a smaller drain and source junction size, and a lower leakage current. A biosensor on SOI requires fewer lithographic steps [52–53]. In our previous work, we proposed a DGDMFET and used virus biomolecules' dielectric constants to demonstrate an SOI FET-based biosensor for detecting the COVID-19 causative virus [54].

In SARS-CoV-2, glycoprotein makes up the virus's S-protein, and the general dielectric constant range for proteins lies in the range between 1 to 4 [55–57]. Therefore, to detect the virus's biomolecules using DMFET, its dielectric constant must be taken in the range of 1 to 4. A significant variation in the drain current by increasing the dielectric constant, confirms that the DMFET can detect virus biomolecules [54].

12.7 CHALLENGES IN BIOSENSING RESEARCH

Biosensors have been in development for almost 50 years, and in the last ten years, this topic has attracted many researchers. However, only a few biosensors are commercially successful [58]. The regulatory terms for clinical applications are extremely complex; one of the factors causing this financial issue. It is challenging to put recent developments and innovations in biosensors into operation. The sensitivity of a biosensor may be affected by non-specific interactions in addition to an actual sample [59]. Controlling antibody and viral binding efficiency might be problematic at times. For effective application in pandemics, optimal biosensor properties must be created. Some characteristics must be considered to achieve good performance and sensitivity; for example, short channel effects must be reduced to improve the performance of FET biosensor devices. Various alternatives, such as SOI FET, are to be employed to minimize short channel effects. A suitable immobilization approach must be utilized for high binding efficiency and low absorption on the biosensor's surface. The correct immobilization approach can increase a sensing device's sensitivity and detection limit [60]. The noise produced by non-targeted biomolecules influences the results of the biosensor, which can be avoided by employing FET devices as biosensors. With the assumption that the biomolecules must fill the cavity formed in the FET device, the device analysis is performed, which impacts sensitivity.

A fully filled cavity with a virus molecule shows more sensitivity than a half-filled or partially filled cavity. Formation of nanogap during fabrication must be carried out in a very concise way [61]. The biosensor components are crucial in increasing the sensitivity of biosensors; for instance, carbon nanotubes (CNTs) can detect proteins, viruses, nucleic acids, antibodies and enzymes [62]. CNTs and graphene enhance the sensitivity by improving the immobilization and adsorption of the enzyme. In the future, consideration of the structural aspect is crucial as adequately designed biosensors can produce accurate results. The biggest challenge is the cost of designing, packaging, testing, manufacturing, industrial processing technique and transportation. If taken care of appropriately, the suggested challenges can provide a superior development opportunity for the new generation of low-cost, extremely sensitive FET-based biosensors.

12.8 CONCLUSION

Since March 2020, the COVID-19 epidemic has dominated the world. Despite medical, hygiene, and healthcare breakthroughs, COVID-19 has emphasized our susceptibility to viral infectious diseases as our greatest problem. In terms of total mortality and socioeconomic effects, COVID-19 has outperformed the ebola epidemic, the influenza (H1N1) pandemic, the Zika epidemic, and the HIV/AIDS global pandemic. This indicates the high requirement and critical role of diagnostics in combating the spread of disease. Over the past few decades, extensive research has been done on the sensitive and selective detection of viruses. DMFET-based biosensing approaches have been preferred over PCR or ELISA because of their quick reaction times, low costs, easy fabrication and minimal sample size requirements. The advancements in FET-based biosensors are the product of multidisciplinary approaches that go above and beyond the usual work. In this chapter, dielectric modulated DGFET has been reviewed to determine whether it is suitable as a biosensing device for detecting the COVID-19 causative virus. Suppose the solutions linked to FET biosensors' commercial cost and reliability factor get adopted realistically and broadly. In that case, point-of-care diagnostics could be a cause of revolution in the healthcare industry. Effective and quick detection will improve the management of pandemics by preventing the spreading of the virus, which will help us prepare for a safe and happy future.

REFERENCES

[1] Santiago, Ibon. "Trends and Innovations in Biosensors for COVID-19 Mass Testing." *ChemBioChem* 21, no. 20 (2020): 2880–89. https://doi.org/10.1002/cbic.202000250.

[2] Fauci, Anthony S., H. Clifford Lane, and Robert R. Redfield. "COVID-19 — Navigating the Uncharted." *New England Journal of Medicine* 382, no. 13 (2020): 1268–69. https://doi.org/10.1056/nejme2002387.

[3] Iravani, Siavash. "Nano- And Biosensors for the Detection of SARS-CoV-2: Challenges and Opportunities." *Materials Advances* 1, no. 9 (2020): 3092–3103. https://doi.org/10.1039/d0ma00702a.

[4] Zhou, Peng, Xing Lou Yang, Xian Guang Wang, Ben Hu, Lei Zhang, Wei Zhang, Hao Rui Si, et al. "A Pneumonia Outbreak Associated with a New Coronavirus of Probable Bat Origin." *Nature* 579, no. 7798 (2020): 270–73. https://doi.org/10.1038/s41586-020-2012-7.

[5] Chorba, Terence. "The Concept of the Crown and Its Potential Role in the Downfall of Coronavirus." *Emerging Infectious Diseases* 26, no. 9 (September 2020): 2302–5. https://doi.org/10.3201/eid2609.AC2609.

[6] Vishwanathan, "All You Need to Know About Coronavirus in India." (2020). https://www.unicef.org/india/coronavirus/covid-19, UNICEF India.

[7] Chamola, Vinay, Vikas Hassija, Vatsal Gupta, and Mohsen Guizani. "A Comprehensive Review of the COVID-19 Pandemic and the Role of IoT, Drones, AI, Blockchain, and 5G in Managing Its Impact." *IEEE Access* 8, no. April (2020): 90225–65. https://doi.org/10.1109/ACCESS.2020.2992341.

[8] Fehr, Anthony R. and Perlman Stanley. "Coronaviruses: An Overview of Their Replication and Pathogenesis." In *Coronaviruses: Methods and Protocols*, 1282:1–282, 2015. https://doi.org/10.1007/978-1-4939-2438-7.

[9] Preparedness, E. "Emergency Preparedness and Response CDC Emergency Operations Center Activations." https://emergency.cdc.gov/recentincidents/index.asp, (2020) 2018–2019.

[10] Zhang, Luoping, and Helen Guo. "Biomarkers of COVID-19 and Technologies to Combat SARS-CoV-2." *Advances in Biomarker Sciences and Technology* 2 (2020): 1–23. https://doi.org/10.1016/j.abst.2020.08.001.

[11] Chan, Jasper Fuk Kin Hang Woo, Zheng Zhu Kok, Hin Chu, Kelvin Kai-Wang To, Shuofeng Yuan, and Kwok Yung Yuen. "Genomic Characterization of the 2019 Novel Human-Pathogenic Coronavirus Isolated from a Patient with Atypical Pneumonia after Visiting Wuhan." *Emerging Microbes and Infections* 9, no. 1 (2020): 221–36. https://doi.org/10.1080/22221751.2020.1719902.

[12] Tan, Yee-Joo, Seng Gee Lim, and Wanjin Hong. "Characterization of Viral Proteins Encoded by the SARS-Coronavirus Genome." *Antiviral Research* 65, no. 2 (2005): 69–78. https://doi.org/10.1016/j.antiviral.2004.10.001.

[13] Siddell, S., H. Wege, and V. Ter Meulen. "The Biology of Coronaviruses." *The Journal of General Virology* 64, no. Pt 4 (1983): 761–76. https://doi.org/10.1099/0022-1317-64-4-761.

[14] Lang, Yifei, Wentao Li, Zeshi Li, Danielle Koerhuis, Arthur C.S. Van Den Burg, Erik Rozemuller, Berend Jan Bosch, et al. "Coronavirus Hemagglutinin-Esterase and Spike Proteins Coevolve for Functional Balance and Optimal Virion Avidity." *Proceedings of the National Academy of Sciences of the United States of America* 117, no. 41 (2020): 25759–70. https://doi.org/10.1073/pnas.2006299117.

[15] Excler, Jean Louis, Melanie Saville, Seth Berkley, and Jerome H. Kim. "Vaccine Development for Emerging Infectious Diseases." *Nature Medicine* 27, no. 4 (2021): 591–600. https://doi.org/10.1038/s41591-021-01301-0.

[16] Keni, Raghuvir, Anila Alexander, Pawan Ganesh Nayak, Jayesh Mudgal, and Krishnadas Nandakumar. "COVID-19: Emergence, Spread, Possible Treatments, and Global Burden." *Frontiers in Public Health* 8 (2020). https://doi.org/10.3389/fpubh.2020.00216.

[17] Smart Detect SARS-CoV-2 rRT-PCR Kit Instructions for Use for Emergency Use Authorization (EUA), pp. 1–18, https://www.fda.gov/media/136786/download.

[18] XPRSARS-COV2–10 302–3562, Rev B April 2020 Instructions for Use For Use Under an Emergency Use Authorization (EUA), pp. Apr. 2020. https://www.fda.gov/media/136314/download.

[19] Wangkheirakpam, Vandana Devi, Brinda Bhowmick, and Puspa Devi Pukhrambam. "Detection of SARS-CoV-2 Using Dielectric Modulated TFET-Based Biosensor." *Journal of Materials Science: Materials in Electronics* 33, no. 13 (2022): 10323–34. https://doi.org/10.1007/s10854-022-08020-3.

[20] Sheikhzadeh, Elham, Shimaa Eissa, Aziah Ismail, and Mohammed Zourob. "Diagnostic Techniques for COVID-19 and New Developments." *Talanta* 220, no. July (2020): 121392. https://doi.org/10.1016/j.talanta.2020.121392.

[21] Petrosillo, N., G. Viceconte, O. Ergonul, G. Ippolito, and E. Petersen. "COVID-19, SARS and MERS: Are They Closely Related?" *Clinical Microbiology and Infection* 26, no. 6 (2020): 729–34. https://doi.org/10.1016/j.cmi.2020.03.026.

[22] Oran, Daniel P., and Eric J. Topol. "Prevalence of Asymptomatic SARS-CoV-2 Infection. A Narrative Review." *Annals of Internal Medicine* 173, no. 5 (2020): 362–68. https://doi.org/10.7326/M20-3012.

[23] Afzal, Adeel. "Molecular Diagnostic Technologies for COVID-19: Limitations and Challenges." *Journal of Advanced Research* 26, no. xxxx (2020): 149–59. https://doi.org/10.1016/j.jare.2020.08.002.

[24] Castillo-Henríquez, Luis, Mariana Brenes-Acuña, Arianna Castro-Rojas, Rolando Cordero-Salmerón, Mary Lopretti-Correa, and José Roberto Vega-Baudrit. "Biosensors for the Detection of Bacterial and Viral Clinical Pathogens." *Sensors (Switzerland)* 20, no. 23 (2020): 1–26. https://doi.org/10.3390/s2023 6926.

[25] Lim, Wei Yin, Boon Leong Lan, and Narayanan Ramakrishnan. "Emerging Biosensors to Detect Severe Acute Respiratory Syndrome Coronavirus 2 (SARS-CoV-2): A Review." *Biosensors* 11, no. 11 (2021): 434.

[26] Bhalla, Nikhil, Pawan Jolly, Nello Formisano, and Pedro Estrela. "Introduction to Biosensors." *Essays in Biochemistry* 60, no. 1 (2016): 1–8. https://doi.org/10.1042/EBC20150001.

[27] Yi, Zhihui, and Jonathan Sayago. "Transistors as an Emerging Platform for Portable Amplified Biodetection in Preventive Personalized Point-of-Care Testing." *Different Types of Field-Effect Transistors – Theory and Applications* (2017). https://doi.org/10.5772/67794.

[28] Soloducho, Jadwiga, and Joanna Cabaj. "Electrochemical and Optical Biosensors in Medical Applications." *Biosensors — Micro and Nanoscale Applications* (2015). https://doi.org/10.5772/60967.

[29] Shrivastav, Anand M., Uroš Cvelbar, and Ibrahim Abdulhalim. "A Comprehensive Review on Plasmonic-Based Biosensors Used in Viral Diagnostics." *Communications Biology* 4, no. 1 (2021): 1–12. https://doi.org/10.1038/s42003-020-01615-8.

[30] Syu, Yu-Cheng, Wei-En Hsu, and Chih-Ting Lin. "Review—Field-Effect Transistor Biosensing: Devices and Clinical Applications." *ECS Journal of*

Solid State Science and Technology 7, no. 7 (2018): Q3196–3207. https://doi. org/10.1149/2.0291807jss.

[31] Sung, Daeun, and Jahyun Koo. "A Review of BioFET's Basic Principles and Materials for Biomedical Applications." *Biomedical Engineering Letters* 11, no. 2 (2021): 85–96. https://doi.org/10.1007/s13534-021-00187-8.

[32] Cho, Il Hoon, Dong Hyung Kim, and Sangsoo Park. "Electrochemical Biosensors: Perspective on Functional Nanomaterials for on-Site Analysis." *Biomaterials Research* 24, no. 1 (2020): 1–12. https://doi.org/10.1186/s40824-019-0181-y.

[33] Grieshaber, Dorothee, Robert MacKenzie, Janos Vörös, and Erik Reimhult. "Electrochemical Biosensors – Sensor Principles and Architectures." *Sensors* 8, no. 3 (2008): 1400–1458. https://doi.org/10.3390/s8031400.

[34] Chen, Chen, and Junsheng Wang. "Optical Biosensors: An Exhaustive and Comprehensive Review." *Analyst* 145, no. 5 (2020): 1605–28. https://doi.org/ 10.1039/c9an01998g.

[35] Sadighbayan, Deniz, Mohammad Hasanzadeh, and Ebrahim Ghafar-Zadeh. "Biosensing Based on Field-Effect Transistors (FET): Recent Progress and Challenges." *TrAC, Trends in Analytical Chemistry* 133 (2020): 116067. https://doi.org/10.1016/j.trac.2020.116067.

[36] Lei, Ka Meng, Pui In Mak, Man Kay Law, and Rui P. Martins. "CMOS Biosensors for: In Vitro Diagnosis-Transducing Mechanisms and Applications." *Lab on a Chip* 16, no. 19 (2016): 3664–81. https://doi.org/10.1039/c6lc01002d.

[37] Pishva, Parsa, and Meral Yüce. "Nanomaterials to Tackle the COVID-19 Pandemic." *Emergent Materials* 4, no. 1 (2021): 211–29. https://doi.org/10. 1007/s42247-021-00184-8.

[38] Asghari, Aref, Chao Wang, Kyoung Min Yoo, Ali Rostamian, Xiaochuan Xu, Jong Dug Shin, Hamed Dalir, and Ray T. Chen. "Fast, Accurate, Point-of-Care COVID-19 Pandemic Diagnosis Enabled through Advanced Lab-on-Chip Optical Biosensors: Opportunities and Challenges." *Applied Physics Reviews* 8, no. 3 (2021). https://doi.org/10.1063/5.0022211.

[39] Kevadiya, Bhavesh D., Jatin Machhi, Jonathan Herskovitz, Maxim D. Oleynikov, Wilson R. Blomberg, Neha Bajwa, Dhruvkumar Soni, et al. "Diagnostics for SARS-CoV-2 Infections." *Nature Materials* 20, no. 5 (2021): 593–605. https://doi.org/10.1038/s41563-020-00906-z.

[40] Makowski, Matthew S., and Albena Ivanisevic. "Molecular Analysis of Blood with Micro-/Nanoscale Field-Effect-Transistor Biosensors." *Small* 7, no. 14 (2011): 1863–75. https://doi.org/10.1002/smll.201100211.

[41] Vu, Cao An, and Wen Yih Chen. "Field-Effect Transistor Biosensors for Biomedical Applications: Recent Advances and Future Prospects." *Sensors (Switzerland)* 19, no. 19 (2019). https://doi.org/10.3390/s19194214.

[42] Reed, Mark A. "CMOS Biosensor Devices and Applications." *Technical Digest - International Electron Devices Meeting, IEDM*, no. 1 (2013): 208–11. https:// doi.org/10.1109/IEDM.2013.6724587.

[43] Fathi-Hafshejani, Parvin, Nurul Azam, Lu Wang, Marcelo A. Kuroda, Michael C. Hamilton, Sahar Hasim, and Masoud Mahjouri-Samani. "Two-Dimensional-Material-Based Field-Effect Transistor Biosensor for Detecting COVID-19 Virus (SARS-CoV-2)." *ACS Nano* 15, no. 7 (2021): 11461–69. https://doi.org/ 10.1021/acsnano.1c01188.

[44] Zamzami, Mazin A., Gulam Rabbani, Abrar Ahmad, Ahmad A. Basalah, Wesam H. Al-Sabban, Saeyoung Nate Ahn, and Hani Choudhry. "Carbon Nanotube

Field-Effect Transistor (CNT-FET)-Based Biosensor for Rapid Detection of SARS-CoV-2 (COVID-19) Surface Spike Protein S1." *Bioelectrochemistry* 143 (2022): 107982. https://doi.org/10.1016/j.bioelechem.2021.107982.

[45] Krsihna, B. Vamsi, Shaik Ahmadsaidulu, Surapaneni Sai Tarun Teja, D. Jayanthi, Alluri Navaneetha, P. Rahul Reddy, and M. Durga Prakash. "Design and Development of Graphene FET Biosensor for the Detection of SARS-CoV-2." *Silicon* (2021). https://doi.org/10.1007/s12633-021-01372-1.

[46] Im, Hyungsoon, Xing Jiu Huang, Bonsang Gu, and Yang Kyu Choi. "A Dielectric-Modulated Field-Effect Transistor for Biosensing." *Nature Nanotechnology* 2, no. 7 (2007): 430–34. https://doi.org/10.1038/nnano.2007.180.

[47] Kim, Sungho, David Baek, Jee Yeon Kim, Sung Jin Choi, Myeong Lok Seol, and Yang Kyu Choi. "A Transistor-Based Biosensor for the Extraction of Physical Properties from Biomolecules." *Applied Physics Letters* 101, no. 7 (2012). https://doi.org/10.1063/1.4745769.

[48] Kim, Chang Hoon, Cheulhee Jung, Hyun Gyu Park, and Yang Kyu Choi. "Novel Dielectric-Modulated Field-Effect Transistor for Label-Free DNA Detection." *Biochip Journal* 2, no. 2 (2009): 127–34.

[49] Das, Amit, S. Rewari, B. K. Kanaujia S. S. Deswal, and R.S. Gupta. "Numerical modeling of a dielectric modulated surrounding-triple-gate germanium-source MOSFET (DM-STGGS-MOSFET)-based biosensor." *J. Comput. Electron* 22, no. 2 (2023): 742–759. https://doi.org/10.1007/s10825-023-02008-w

[50] Das, Rahul, Ankush Chattopadhyay, Manash Chanda, Chandan K. Sarkar, and Chayanika Bose. "Analytical Modeling of Sensitivity Parameters Influenced by Practically Feasible Arrangement of Bio-Molecules in Dielectric Modulated FET Biosensor." *Silicon*, 14, no. 15 (2022): 9417–9430. https://doi.org/10.1007/s12633-021-01617-z.

[51] Yadav, Shivendra, Anju Gedam, and Sukeshni Tirkey. "A Dielectric Modulated Biosensor for SARS-CoV-2." *IEEE Sensors Journal* 21, no. 13 (2021): 14483–90. https://doi.org/10.1109/JSEN.2020.3019036.

[52] Chan, Mansun, Fariborz Assaderaghi, Chenming Hu, Ping K. Ko, and Stephen A. Parke. "Recessed-Channel Structure for Fabricating Ultrathin SOI MOSFET with Low Series Resistance." *IEEE Electron Device Letters* 15, no. 1 (1994): 22–24. https://doi.org/10.1109/55.289474.

[53] Koh, Yo Hwan, JinHyeok Choi, Myung Hee Nam, and Ji Woon Yang. "Body-Contacted SOI MOSFET Structure with Fully Bulk CMOS Compatible Layout and Process." *IEEE Electron Device Letters* 18, no. 3 (1997): 102–4. https://doi.org/10.1109/55.556094.

[54] Kumar, Saurabh, R. K. Chauhan, and Manish Kumar. "Sensitivity Enhancement of Dual Gate FET Based Biosensor Using Modulated Dielectric for Covid Detection." *Silicon* (2022). https://doi.org/10.1007/s12633-022-01865-7.

[55] Parihar, Mukta Singh, and Abhinav Kranti. "Enhanced Sensitivity of Double Gate Junctionless Transistor Architecture for Biosensing Applications." *Nanotechnology* 26, no. 14 (2015): 145201. https://doi.org/10.1088/0957-4484/26/14/145201.

[56] Talley, Kemper, Carmen Ng, Michael Shoppell, Petras Kundrotas, and Emil Alexov. "On the Electrostatic Component of Protein-Protein Binding Free Energy." *PMC Biophysics* 1, no. 1 (2008): 1–23. https://doi.org/10.1186/1757-5036-1-2.

[57] Gilson, Michael K., and Barry H. Honig. "The Dielectric Constant of a Folded Protein." *Biopolymers* 25, no. 11 (1986): 2097–2119. https://doi.org/10.1002/bip.360251106.

[58] Zhang, Lulu, Wenqiong Su, Shuopeng Liu, Chengjie Huang, Behafarid Ghalandari, Adeleh Divsalar, and Xianting Ding. "Recent Progresses in Electrochemical DNA Biosensors for MicroRNA Detection." *Phenomics* 2, no. 1 (2022): 18–32. https://doi.org/10.1007/s43657-021-00032-z.

[59] Naresh, Varnakavi, and Nohyun Lee. "A Review on Biosensors and Recent Development of Nanostructured Materials-Enabled Biosensors." *Sensors (Switzerland)* 21, no. 4 (2021): 1–35. https://doi.org/10.3390/s21041109.

[60] Shoorideh, Kaveh, and Chi On Chui. "On the Origin of Enhanced Sensitivity in Nanoscale FET-Based Biosensors." *Proceedings of the National Academy of Sciences of the United States of America* 111, no. 14 (2014): 5111–16. https://doi.org/10.1073/pnas.1315485111.

[61] Wadhera, Tanu, Deepti Kakkar, Girish Wadhwa, and Balwinder Raj. "Recent Advances and Progress in Development of the Field Effect Transistor Biosensor: A Review." *Journal of Electronic Materials* 48, no. 12 (2019): 7635–46. https://doi.org/10.1007/s11664-019-07705-6.

[62] Capek, I. *Carbon Nanotubes-Growth and Applications*, ed. M. Naraghi (Rijeka: IntechOpen, 2011), p. 75.

Chapter 13

Integration of Artificial Intelligence with Opto-VLSI for the Biomedical and Healthcare Industries

Jyoti Kandpal

Graphic Era (deemed to be a University), Uttarakhand, India

Geetanjali Baluti

THDC Institute of Hydropower Engineering and Technology, Uttarakhand, India

Praful Ranjan

Government Girls Polytechnic, Varanasi, India

CONTENTS

ABBREVIATIONS

AI	Artificial Intelligence
AN	Artificial network
ANN	Artificial neural networks
BPNN	Back propagation neural network
CAD	Computer-aided design
CB	ChubbyBrain
CBR	Case-based reasoning
CMOS	Complementary metal oxide semiconductor
CNN	Convolutional neural networks
CT	Computed tomography

DOI: 10.1201/9781003431138-13

DARPA	Defense advanced research projects agency
DNN	Deep neural network
ECG	Electrocardiogram
EDA	Electronic design automation
FET	Field effect transistor
GBR	Gradient boosting
GNN	Graph neural network
GPR	Gaussian process regression
GRAIDS	Gastrointestinal artificial intelligence diagnostic system
HBM	High bandwidth memory
IC	Integrated circuit
KNN	K-nearest neighbor
LR	Linear regression
MARS	Multivariate adaptive regression splines
ML	Machine Learning
MLP	Multilayer perceptron
MR	Multiple regression
NCR	National capital region
PCA	Principal component analysis
PCB	Printed circuitboard
PPA	Power, performance and area
RBF	Radial basis function
RISC	Reduced instruction set compute
RL	Reinforcement learning
RNN	Recurrent neural network
SoC	System on chip
SVM	Support vector machines
SVR	Support vector regression
VGG	Visual geometry group
VLSI	Very large scale integration
WEKA	Waikato Environment for Knowledge Analysis

13.1 INTRODUCTION

The introduction of complementary metal-oxide-semiconductor (CMOS) transistors in the integrated circuit (IC) sector prompted a dramatic shift in the field of electronics, beginning in the era of semiconductor technology. CMOS technology has since become the industry standard in the realm of microelectronics. Since the 1960s, the transistor count on a single chip has expanded exponentially [1, 2]. Over many technical generations, continual downscaling of transistors has improved performance and density [3], resulting in remarkable growth in the microelectronics sector – modern, very large-scale integration (VLSI) technology. The rising demand for power-sensitive designs with advanced features has resulted from the high demand for portable gadgets in recent years. Highly advanced and scalable VLSI circuits are meeting the ever-increasing demand in the microelectronics sector. Compatible device downscaling, which results in improved device performance, is one of the primary factors accelerating advancements in IC technology. Devices are currently being scaled down to sub-3nm gates and beyond. However, the increasingly downscaling CMOS technology has given device engineers a lot of fresh challenges and prospects. As transistor size shrinks, the semiconductor process becomes more complex. Simple scaling eventually stops as we get closer to atomic dimensions.

Even though devices are small, several performance aspects deteriorate, including gain, leakage and sensitivity to manufacturing changes [4–8]. Furthermore, the dramatic enhancement in process variables substantially impacts circuit operation, resulting in varying performance in transistors of the same size. This impacts the circuit's propagation delay, which behaves like a stochastic random variable, confounding timing-closure approaches and negatively reducing chip yield [8]. One of the leading causes of parametric yield loss is increasing process variability in the nanoscale regime. Multigate field-effect transistors (FETs) [9] are more process-variation tolerant than CMOS transistors technology. On the other hand, aggressive scaling impacts their performance parameters [10, 11].

Advanced design approaches and economical design is used to achieve good optimization in the VLSI system. The performance of electronic design automation (EDA) technology is to overcome design constraints on chip turnaround time. Conventional EDA methods take a longer time to find the optimized solution for a design. Additionally, conventional methods are resource and time-intensive, due to delays in time-to-market.

As depicted in Figure 13.1, computer-aided design (CAD) tools are employed at various stages of the chip design cycle, from circuit description to layout design. CAD tools are used to implement and evaluate the performance of highly complicated digital and analog ICs. With the massive increase in transistors per chip, improvising VLSI–CAD tools are becoming increasingly complex and sophisticated. At various stages of VLSI design and manufacture, there are numerous possibilities for developing/integrating ML/AI solutions, enabling accelerated semiconductor and EDA technology convergence. [13, 14].

"Artificial" signifies human-made objects instead of naturally occurring, and "Intelligence" is the ability to learn and create strategies to achieve goals by direct interaction with information. As a result, an intelligent entity must be able to attain knowledge in many different ways, such as through observations, understanding through experiences, analyzing and comprehending information and interacting with others. Furthermore, it should be able to use this acquired knowledge to build conclusions, summarize data, develop and achieve goals, recognize words and pictures and so on.

A machine would mimic human behavior according to a technology known as artificial intelligence (AI). Table 13.1 gives an overview of AI techniques.

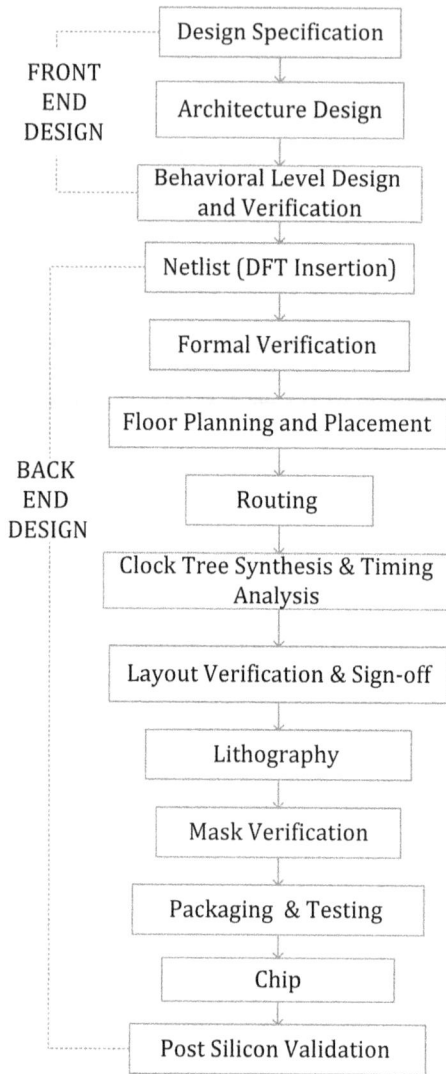

Figure 13.1 Design flow of VLSI technology.

There are two subgroups of AI: deep learning and machine learning. Machine learning (ML) allows systems to learn from previous data without explicitly programming it. Deep learning is the most critical subset of machine learning. When new data is provided, ML incorporates learning and self-correction. AI can process unstructured, semi-structured and structured data compared to ML, which can only process structured and semi-structured data.

Artificial Intelligence is in high demand for semiconductor design and verification, which are now the most demanding tasks. With the rise of

Table 13.1 Overview of liquid and gaseous fuels generated from lignocellulose and their properties

S.No.	Different Abstraction Level	Characteristic	AI/ML Algorithms	CAD/VLSI Tool
1.	Logic Design	Design specification Architectural design Behavioral level design and Verification	Logic Regression Graph Neural Network (GNN) Linear Regression, Ridge Regression Gradient Boosting (GBR), Deep Neural Network (DNN) Multilayer Perceptron (MLP), Convolutional Neural Networks (CNN), K-means (Clusters), K-Nearest Neighbors (KNN), Support Vector Machines (SVM)	Synopsys, Xilinx Cadence Virtuoso
2.	Logic Synthesis	Netlist Formal Verification	KNN, Bayesian network, K-means (Clusters), Linear Regression (LR), Support Vector Regression (SVR), Gaussian Process Regression (GPR), Artificial Neural Networks (ANN), SVM	Synopsys Design Compiler, Cadence Genus
3.	Physical Design	Placement and Floor Planning Routing Clock Tree Synthesis and Timing Analysis, Layout Verification and Sign off	SVM, ANN, Reinforcement learning (RL) Data Mining Tool Multilayer Perceptron (MLP), Random Forest (RF), Multivariate Adaptive Regression Splines (MARS), LR	Synopsis IC Complier, Cadence Innvous
4.	Fabrication	Lithography Mask Verification Packaging and Testing Chip Post Silicon Validation	MLP, High Bandwidth Memory (HBM), SVM, Logistic Regression, Decision Tree, ANN, Modified Naïve Bayes, Deep Learning	Alliance Magic Electric Spyglass DFT, Synopsys Teramax
5.	Testing	Functional Verification Fault Diagnosis Scan Chain Diagnosis	A Bayesian network, K-means clustering MLP, Principal Component Analysis (PCA), Bayesian model	

open-source architectures like RISC V and the abundance of CAD tools for design and verification, a feasible design requires a lot of rendering and testing. Creating and troubleshooting the issues with such a remote workforce will take months. Furthermore, modern chipsets are so vast and sophisticated that designing them manually is time-consuming. Over time, they have been mechanized, utilizing AI design methodologies included in design software.

The semiconductor sector requires a large human workforce and a significant amount of time to design efficient chips. Furthermore, every year, the semiconductor industry expands by introducing new, more efficient technological nodes following market trends. Because of this, it is imperative to accelerate the design cycle time so that the chip design for the current technology node can be created before the next technology node hits the market. If not, the design can become outmoded as soon as the new technical node hits the market. Semi-automating or automating the design cycle is fundamental to minimizing human efforts while maintaining the throughput required for semiconductor designs. The semiconductor design cycle can be optimized substantially better by using AI and ML.

Many sources state that AI has produced prominent answers to various challenges. AI is built on human intelligence that has been interpreted so that a computer can readily duplicate it and do tasks of varying complexity. Furthermore, AI can quickly spot patterns and trends in massive amounts of data, allowing users to make informed decisions. At high computational rates, AI systems can handle multidimensional and multivariate data. These algorithms acquire insight through time, increasing the precision and effectiveness of their predictions. Additionally, they facilitate decision-making by expediting the necessary procedures. Due to the numerous advantages of AI algorithms, their use is increasing in popularity, and AI techniques have been widely applied in the VLSI industry.

13.2 ARTIFICIAL INTELLIGENCE WITH VLSI (AI AND VLSI)

Kirk [15] was the first to explain the influence of AI on VLSI design in 1985. His work outlines the extent and importance of the AI approach in CAD tools at various abstraction stages of the VLSI project. On the other hand, Rabbat and Khan et al debated the benefits of introducing AI into the VLSI design process and its applications [16, 17]. Furthermore, they concentrated on various AI applications for IC production, notably for expert systems as several knowledge-based systems, and NCR design mentors, are employed in the VLSI sector.

In response to significant advancements in AI/ML, researchers have made different pioneering attempts to implement, develop and organize learning approaches to VLSI design and production, as shown in Figure 13.2.

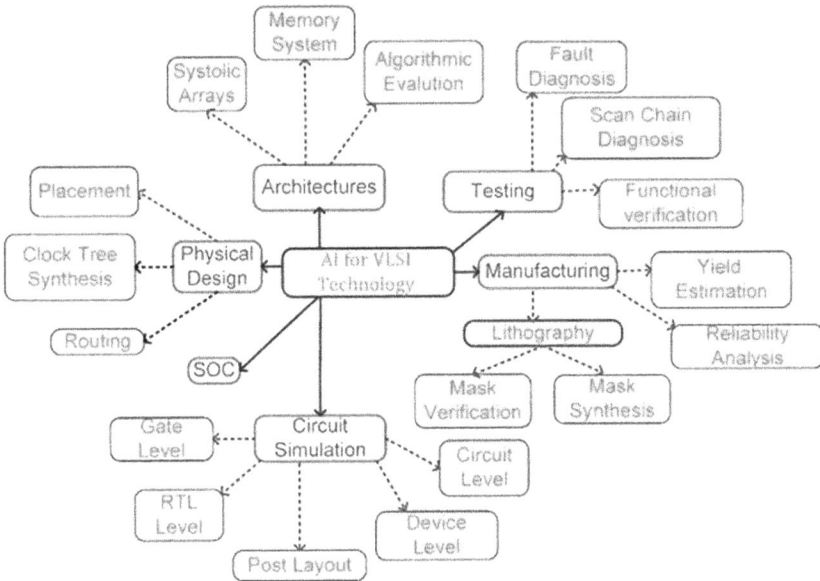

Figure 13.2 Different areas of VLSI technology for considering AI/ML.

These artificial learning algorithms are built and guided with practical, automated technology to enable chip production to turn around rather quickly. We have especially highlighted how ML and AI might be used to enhance chip design to explain how various learning strategies may be implemented.

In 2018, the defense Advanced Research Projects Agency (DARPA) provided funding for the electronic assets (IDEA) effort, which aims to develop a layout generator for System-on-Chip (SoC) with a 24-hour turnaround and "no human in the loop". As a result, we've demonstrated a variety of AI and machine learning strategies for improving the design cycle. Table 13.1 surveys various AI/ML techniques at the VLSI abstraction level.

Electronic design automation (EDA) tools from vendors like Synopsis and Cadence readily adopt machine learning-based methodologies for more efficient design simulation, hence improving the three Ps norm of "Performance, Power, and Price". The EDA companies employ ML analytics and optimization to automate device routing and tuning to improve circuit performance, reliability, resilience, as well as power, performance and area (PPA) outcomes. Moreover, their programs will accelerate the timeline for implementing intelligent design flows to achieve the next significant leap in design productivity.

These activities will improve the range of analog, digital, verification, package and Printed Circuit Board (PCB) EDA technologies, allowing us to provide the most advanced solution to our customers. In addition, these approaches will improve our customers' access to the most modern system design enablement solutions across the whole spectrum of digital analog, package, verification and PCB EDA technologies.

13.3 AI APPLICATIONS IN THE HEALTHCARE AND BIOMEDICAL FIELDS

According to a 2016 survey from CB Insights, artificial intelligence technology is used by 86 per cent of healthcare provider organizations, life science enterprises and healthcare technology vendors. Furthermore, the survey predicted that these companies would average $54 million on artificial intelligence initiatives by 2020.

Rather than totally replacing the work of physicians and other healthcare professionals, AI techniques are commonly employed to improve human work. Artificial intelligence may help healthcare personnel with various tasks, such as administrative work, clinical documentation and patient communication, as well as offering expert support in areas such as patient monitoring, image analysis and medical device automation.

13.4 THE DISTRIBUTION OF PUBLICATIONS FOR DISEASE DIAGNOSIS USING AI APPROACHES

The critical disease areas where AI has been used include cancer, cardiology and neurology. Clinical studies can take years, if not decades, to complete and are incredibly costly. As a result, the fundamental goal of AI startups is to make the process faster and less expensive. As a result, AI in biomedical engineering offers a wide range of applications. AI can also help with tedious, repetitive tasks. Data input, computed tomography (CT) scans, interpreting various tests, X-ray scans, and other jobs can all be done more quickly and accurately by robots. Large volumes of data can be time-consuming and difficult to handle in cardiology and radiology, for example. Table 13.2 displays authors' techniques for detecting various diseases and the accuracy percentages.

With brief innovations in VLSI, computer hardware, and AI, it's feasible to expect VLSI design tools to perform better than humans. It's realistic to believe that a computer will someday be able to evaluate complex trade-offs and choose the optimal design from a vast selection. In addition, a more powerful programming paradigm allows for the creation of more powerful tools. In the long term, synthesis tools such as a complete general-purpose silicon compiler will emerge. This technology will drastically reduce VLSI design timeframes by exploiting scarce engineering resources.

Smartphones with exceptional abilities to understand human speech and respond with appropriate and precise responses, personal devices for smart homes and healthcare and embedded intelligent systems in self-driving cars

Table 13.2 Different disease detection using AI/ML techniques [18]

Reference	Disease	Algorithm	Accuracy
[36] Khan et al. (2020)	Alzheimer's disease	ML, Pipeline, Pattern Recognition	86.84%
[19] Janghel et al. (2020)	Alzheimer's disease	SVM, KNN, Decision Tree	73.46%
[20] Oh et al. (2019)	Alzheimer's disease	Convolution Neural Network (CNN)	86.60%
[21] Jo et al. (2019)	Alzheimer's disease	Recurrent Neural Network (RNN), CNN	96.00%
[22] Plawaik et al. (2018)	Arrhythmia disease	ECG signal, Deep genetic ensemble of classifiers	99.37%
[23] Memon et al. (2019)	Breast cancer	SVM, Machine Learning	99%
[24] Sivakami (2015)	Breast Cancer	Decision Tree, SVM	91%
[25] Venkatesan et al. (2015)	Breast Cancer	Decision Tree	97%
[26] Ahmed (2017)	Cardiac Arrest	KNN, IoT, Machine learning,	96%
[27] Nashif et al. (2018)	Cardiovascular disease	Machine Learning, Data Mining, Waikato Environment for Knowledge Analysis(WEKA), SVM	97.53%
[28] Battineni et al. (2020)	Chronic disease	SVM, Logistic Regression	73.1–91.6%
[29] Aldhyani et al. (2020)	Chronic disease	SVM, KNN, NB, Random Forest	80.55%
[30] Ani et al. (2017)	Chronic disease	Random forest, Naïve Bayes, KNN, Classification	93%
[31] Vasal et al. (2020)	COVID-19 disease	Deep Learning models, VGG16 (Visual Geometry Group), DenseNet121, ResNet50	98.80%
[32] Nazir et.al (2019)	Diabetic Retinopathy	Content Based Image Retrieval	99.60%
[33] Kaur and Kumari (2018)	Diabetic disease	KNN, ANN, multifactor, dimensionality reduction, Radial Basis Function (RBF), SVM	SVM: 0.89 KNN: 0.88 ANN: 0.86 MDR: 0.83
[34] Swapna et al. (2018)	Diabetic disease	CNN, Long Short-Term Memory, SVM,	95.70%
[35] Lukmanto et al. (2015)	Diabetic disease	Fuzzy support vector machine, SVM	89.02%

(Continued)

Table 13.2 (Continued) Different disease detection using AI/ML techniques [18]

Reference	Disease	Algorithm	Accuracy
[36] Khan et al. (2020)	Gastrointestinal disease	VGG 16, ANN, Deep Learning	98.40%
[37]Luo et al. (2019)	Gastrointestinal cancer	GRAIDS (Gastrointestinal Artificial Intelligence Diagnostic System), Clopper Pearson Method	95%
[38] Isravel et al. (2020)	Heart disease	KNN, Naïve Bayes, Decision Tree, ECG signals	80%
[39] Kanegae et al.. (2020)	Hypertension disease	XGBoost, Ensemble, logistic regression	XGBoost: 0.877 Ensemble: 0.881 Logistic Regression: 0.859
[40] Arsalan et al. (2019)	Hypertension disease	Vess-net Method, AI, Semantic Segmentation	96.55%
[41] Nithya et al. (2020)	Kidney disease	K-means clustering, Linear and quadratic-based segmentation, ANN	99.61%
[42] Das et al. (2019)	Liver cancer	Gaussian Mixture Model, DNN classifier	99.38%
[43] Musleh et al. (2019)	Liver disease	ANN model	99%
[44] Chuang et al. (2011)	Liver disease	Case-based reasoning (CBR), Backpropagation Neural Network (BPNN), Logistic Regression, Classification	95%
[45] Romanini et al. (2020)	Oral cancer	ANN, Fuzzy logic	78.89%
[46] Morabito et al. (2016)	Scalp disease	Deep Learning, Convolution neural network (CNN), MLP	80%
[47] Naseer et al. (2019)	Skin disease	MLP, ANN	76.67%
[48] Rodrigues et al. (2020)	Skin disease	CNN, VGG Net, KNN, SVM, Random Forest	96.81%
[49] Hosseinzadeh et al. (2020)	Thyroid disease	ANN	99%
[50] Yadav et al. (2020)	Thyroid disease	Decision Tree, Random Forest, classification, regression tree	Decision tree: 98% Random forest: 99%
[51] Bhatt et al. (2019)	Thyroid disease	ANN, Random Forest, Multiple Regression (MR)	98.22%

(Continued)

Table 13.2 (Continued) Different disease detection using AI/ML techniques [18]

Reference	Disease	Algorithm	Accuracy
[52] Lai et al. (2020)	Tuberculosis	ANN, Random Forest	88.67%
[53] Gao et al. (2019)	Tuberculosis	Deep Learning, ResNet	85.29%
[54] Naser and Naseer (2019)	Tumor detection	Multilayer Perceptron, ANN	76.67%
[55] Chen et al. (2019a, b)	Urology disease	ML, Cox Regression, NN, Decision support system	71.80%

are just a few instances of how current AI is facilitating our lives. Hardware limits, on the other hand, are currently impeding AI progress. For example, embedded electronics, such as sensors and telephones, require low power, but today's processors are frequently power consumers. In addition, sights, sounds and speech must also be classified quickly and accurately. As a result, current CMOS hardware has difficulty balancing low-power and high-speed goals.

13.5 OPTOELECTRONICS WITH VLSI

Photonic devices and VLSI electronics are intimately integrated into OPTOELECTRONIC-VLSI (OE-VLSI) technology. The aim is to develop high-performance VLSI circuits with optical inputs and output signals that can handle data speeds up to and beyond a terabit per second. The OE-VLSI technologies are most successful in systems where high-bandwidth "information" must be received, converted or rapidly evaluated by the electronic circuit and transferred out of the subsystem. This technology provides a significant gain in integration density over all-electrical systems. Furthermore, using OE-VLSI "packaging" reduces (and in some cases eliminates) parasitic associated with traditional packaging technology that uses wire bonds between chips, resulting in a reduction in the energy required to transmit digital signals within the system (and thus the system's power-delay product).

13.6 CHALLENGES IN THE HEALTHCARE AND BIOMEDICAL INDUSTRIES USING AI

The biomedical and healthcare industries face several challenges when using AI:

- Regulatory bodies have provided insufficient clarity on the actions required for regulatory approval.

- AI approaches must either function alongside or replace conventional healthcare workflows. In addition, updated or new workflows in the clinical setting must be validated for accuracy and reproducibility under realistic circumstances and recorded, as well as staff training.
- There is a lack of user-friendly software to let people employ AI in biomedical and healthcare settings.
- The robustness of AI models is poor.

13.7 CONCLUSION

The geometry of the transistor is getting smaller as the performance of semiconductor designs improves, and the technology is moving from simple transistors to non-planar FinFET devices. The Very Large-Scale Integration (VLSI) sector has begun implementing artificial intelligence (AI) techniques in design automation to change the entire chip design methodology. It has been observed that in System-On-Chip (SoC), there is a requirement to decrease the current power consumption of the hardware to integrate ML algorithms to boost its efficiency. As a result, AI is now a crucial component of the VLSI business. In this context, a thorough analysis of numerous aspects of VLSI-related AI has been done. This chapter examines the VLSI design and AI sectors; AI will considerably impact how VLSI design is now carried out. Many human design chores will be automated, leaving designers to work on the most challenging and obscure design issues. These breakthroughs will cover the path for powerful computing hardware and AI research developments.

REFERENCES

1. Carballo J.-A., Chan W.-T. J., Gargini P. A., Kahng A. B., and Nath S. "ITRS 2.0: Toward a re-framing of the semiconductor technology roadmap." In *2014 IEEE 32nd International Conference on Computer Design (ICCD)*, pp. 139–146. IEEE, (2014).
2. Moore G. E. "Cramming more components onto integrated circuits." *In Electronics* 38, no. 8 (1965): 114–117.
3. Wong H.-S. P., David J. F., Solomon P. M., Wann C. H. J., and Welser J. J. "Nanoscale CMOS." *Proceedings of the IEEE* 87, no. 4 (1999): 537–570.
4. Vaddi R., Dasgupta S., and Agarwal R. P. "Device and circuit design challenges in the digital subthreshold region for ultralow-power applications." In *VLSI Design 2009*, 2009.
5. Sylvester D., and Kaul H. "Power-driven challenges in nanometer design." *IEEE Design & Test of Computers* 18, no. 6 (2001): 12–21.
6. Iwai H. "Logic LSI technology roadmap for 22 nm and beyond." In *2009 16th IEEE International Symposium on the Physical and Failure Analysis of Integrated Circuits*, pp. 7–10. IEEE, 2009.

7. Calhoun B. H., Cao Y., Li X., Mai K., Pileggi L. T., Rutenbar R. A., and Shepard K. L.. "Digital circuit design challenges and opportunities in the era of nanoscale CMOS." *Proceedings of the IEEE* 96, no. 2 (2008): 343–365.

8. Abu-Rahma M. H., and Anis M. "Variability in VLSI circuits: Sources and design considerations." In *2007 IEEE International Symposium on Circuits and Systems*, pp. 3215–3218. IEEE, 2007.

9. Chaudhuri S., and Jha N. K. "FinFET logic circuit optimization with different FinFET styles: Lower power possible at higher supply voltage." In *2014 27th International Conference on VLSI Design and 2014 13th International Conference on Embedded Systems*, pp. 476–482. IEEE, 2014.

10. Rathore R. S., Rana A. K., and Sharma R. "Threshold voltage variability induced by statistical parameters fluctuations in nanoscale bulk and SOI FinFETs." In *2017 4th International Conference on Signal Processing, Computing and Control (ISPCC)*, pp. 377–380. IEEE, 2017.

11. Brown A. R., Daval N., Bourdelle K. K., Nguyen B.-Y., and Asenov A. "Comparative simulation analysis of process-induced variability in nanoscale SOI and bulk trigate FinFETs." *IEEE Transactions on Electron Devices* 60, no. 11 (2013): 3611–3617.

12. Belleville M., Thomas O., Valentian A., and Clermidy F. "Designing digital circuits with nanoscale devices: Challenges and opportunities." *Solid-State Electronics* 84 (2013): 38–45.

13. Wang L., and Luo M. "Machine learning applications and opportunities in IC design flow." In *2019 International Symposium on VLSI Design, Automation and Test (VLSI-DAT)*, pp. 1–3. IEEE, 2019.

14. Lee C.-K. "Deep Learning Creativity in EDA." In *2020 International Symposium on VLSI Design, Automation and Test (VLSI-DAT)*, pp. 1–1. IEEE, 2020.

15. Kirk R. S. "The impact of AI technology on VLSI design." In *Managing Requirements Knowledge, International Workshop on*, pp. 125–125. IEEE Computer Society, 1985.

16. Rabbat G. "VLSI and AI are getting closer." *IEEE circuits and Devices Magazine* 4, no. 1 (1988): 15–18.

17. Khan M. Z. A., Saleem H., and Afzal S.. "Application of VLSI in artificial intelligence." *International Organization for Scientific Research-IOSR Journal of Computer Engineering (IOSR-JCE)* 6, no. 2 (2012): 23–25.

18. Kumar Y., Koul A., Singla R., and Ijaz M. F. "Artificial intelligence in disease diagnosis: A systematic literature review, synthesizing framework and future research agenda." *Journal of Ambient Intelligence and Humanized Computing*, 29 (2022): 1–28.

19 Janghel R.R., and Rathore Y.K. "Deep convolution neural network-based system for early diagnosis of Alzheimer's disease." *Irbm* (2020) 1:1–10.

20. Oh K., Chung Y.C., Kim K.W., Kim W.S., and Oh I.S. "Classification and visualization of Alzheimer's disease using volumetric convolutional neural network and transfer learning." *Sci Rep* 9 (2019).

21. Jo T., Nho K., and Saykin A.J. "Deep learning in Alzheimer's disease: diagnostic classification and prognostic prediction using neuroimaging data." *Front Aging Neurosci* (2019).

22. Plawiak P., Ozal Y., Tan R., and Acharya U. "Arrhythmia detection using deep convolution neural network with long duration ECG signals." *Comput Biol Med* (2018) 102: 411–420.

23. Memon M., Li J., Haq A., and Memon M. "Breast cancer detection in the IoT health environment using modified recursive feature selection." *Wirel Commun Mob* (2019):19.

24. Sivakami, K., and Saraswathi, N. "Mining big data: breast cancer prediction using DT-SVM hybrid model." *International Journal of Scientific Engineering and Applied Science (IJSEAS)*, (2015). 1(5): 418–429.

25. Venkatesan, E. V., and Velmurugan, T. "Performance analysis of decision tree algorithms for breast cancer classification." *Indian Journal of Science and Technology*, (2015) 8(29): 1–8.

26. Ahmed F. "An Internet of Things (IoT) application for predicting the quantity of future heart attack patients." *J Comput Appl* (2017) 164: 36–40.

27. Nashif S., Raihan R., Islam R., Imam M.H., "Heart disease detection by using machine learning algorithms and a real-time cardiovascular health monitoring system." *HealthcTechnol* (2018) 6: 854–8.

28. Battineni G., Sagaro G.G., Chinatalapudi N., Amenta F. "Applications of machine learning predictive models in the chronic disease diagnosis." *J Personal Med* (2020).

29. Aldhyani T.H.H., Alshebami A.S., and Alzahrani M.Y. "Soft clustering for enhancing the diagnosis of chronic diseases over machine learning algorithms." *J Healthc Eng* (2020).

30. Ani R., Krishna S., Anju N., Aslam M.S., and Deepa O.S. "IoT based patient monitoring and diagnostic prediction tool using ensemble classifier." In: *2017 International conference on advances in computing, communications and informatics (ICACCI)*, (2017) pp. 1588–1593.

31. Vasal S., Jain S., and Verma A. "COVID-AI: an artificial intelligence system to diagnose COVID-19 disease." *J Eng Res Technol* (2020) 9: 1–6.

32. Nazir T., Irtaza A., Shabbir Z., Javed A., Akram U., and Tariq M "Artificial intelligence in medicine diabetic retinopathy detection through novel tetragonal local octa patterns and extreme learning machines." *Artif Intell Med* (2019) 99:101695.

33. Kaur H., and Kumari V. "Predictive modelling and analytics for diabetes using a machine learning approach." *Appl Comput Inf* (2018).

34. Swapna G., Vinayakumar R., and Soman K.P. "Diabetes detection using deep learning algorithms." *ICT Express* (2018) 4: 243–246.

35. Lukwanto R., and Irwansyah E. "The early detection of diabetes mellitus using fuzzy hierarchical model." *Proc Comput Sci* (2015) 59: 312–31.

36. Khan A., Khan M., Ahmed F., Mittal M., Goyal L., Hemanth D., and Satapathy S. "Gastrointestinal diseases segmentation and classifcation based on duo-deep architectures." *Pattern Recognit Lett.* (2020) 131: 193–204.

37. Luo, Xin, Ying Wang, Yue Hao, Xing-ji Li, Chao-Ming Liu, Xin-Xing Fei, Cheng-Hao Yu, and Fei Cao. "Research of single-event burnout and hardening of AlGaN/GaN-based MISFET." *IEEE Transactions on Electron Devices* 66, no. 2 (2019): 1118–1122.

38. Isravel D.P., and Silas S.V.P.D. "Improved heart disease diagnostic IoT model using machine learning techniques." *Neuroscience* (2020) 9:4442–4446.

39. Kanegae H., Suzuki K., Fukatani K., Ito T., Kairo K., and Beng N. "Highly precise risk prediction model for new onset hypertension using artificial neural network techniques." *J Clin Hypertens* (2020) 22: 445–450.

40. Arsalan M., Owasis M., Mahmood T., Cho S., and Park K. "Aiding the diagnosis of diabetic and hypertensive retinopathy using artificial intelligence based semantic segmentation." *J Clin Med* (2019) 8:1446.
41. Nithya A., Ahilan A., Venkatadri N., Ramji D., and Palagan A. "Kidney disease detection and segmentation using artificial neural network and multi kernel k-means clustering for ultrasound images." *Measurement* (2020) 149:106952.
42. Das A., Acharya U.R., Panda S.S., and Sabut S. "Deep learning based liver cancer detection using watershed transform and Gaussian mixture model techniques." *Cogn Syst* (2019) 54:165–175.
43. Musleh M., Alajrami E., Khalil A., Nasser B., Barhoom A., and Naser S. "Predicting liver patients using artificial neural network." *J Acad Inf Syst Res* (2019) 3: 1–11
44. Chuang C. "Case based reasoning support for liver disease diagnosis." *Artif Intell* (2011) 53: 15–23.
45. Romanini J., Barun L., Martins M., and Carrard V. "Continuing education activities improve dentists self-efficacy to manage oral mucosal lesions and oral cancer." *Eur J Dent Educ* (2020) 25: 28–34
46. Morabito F., Campolo M., Leracitano C., Ebadi J., Bonanno L., Barmanti A., Desalvo S., Barmanti P., and Ieracitano C. "Deep Convolutional neural Network for classifcation of mild cognitive impaired and Alzheimer's disease patients from scalp EEG recordings." *Res Technol Soc Ind Levaraging Better Tomorrow* (2016).
47. Naser S., and Naseer I. "Lung cancer detection using artificial neural network." *J Eng Inf Sys Res t* (2019) 3:17–23.
48. Rodrigues D.A., Ivo R.F., Satapathy S.C., Wang S., Hemanth J., and Filo P.P.R. "A new approach for classification skin lesion based on transfer learning, deep learning, and IoT system." *Pattern Recognit Lett* (2020) 136: 8–15.
49. Hosseinzadeh M., Ahmed O., Ghafour M., Safara F., Ali S., Vo B., and Chiang H. "A multiple multilayer perceptron neural network with an adaptive learning algorithm for thyroid disease diagnosis in the internet of medical things." *J Supercomput.* (2020) https://doi.org/10.1007/s11227-020-03404-w
50. Yadav D., and Pal S. "Prediction of thyroid disease using decision tree ensemble method." *Hum Intell Syst Integr.* (2020) https://doi.org/10.1007/s42454-020-00006-y
51. Bhatt V., and Pal V. "An intelligent system for diagnosing thyroid disease in pregnant ladies through artificial neural network." In: *Conference on advances in engineering science management and technology*, (2019) pp. 1–10.
52. Lai N., Shen W., Lee C., Chang J., Hsu M. et al "Comparison of the predictive outcomes for anti-Alzheimer drug-induced hepatotoxicity by different machine learning techniques." *Comput Methods Programs Biomed* (2020) 188: 105307.
53. Zhou Z., Yang L., Gao J., and Chen X. "Structure–relaxivity relationships of magnetic nanoparticles for magnetic resonance imaging." *Adv Mater* (2019) 31: 1804567.
54. Nasser I., Naser S. et al "Predicting tumor category using artificial neural network." *Eng Inf Technol* (2019) 3:1–7.
55. Chen J., Remulla D., Nguyen J., Aastha D., Liu Y., and Dasgupta P. "Current status of artificial intelligence applications in urology and their potential to influence clinical practice." *BJU Int* (2019a, b) 124: 567–577.

Chapter 14

VLSI Computer Aided Design Using Machine Learning for Biomedical Applications

Karan Singh and Shruti Kalra

Jaypee Institute of Information Technology, Noida, Uttar Pradesh, India

CONTENTS

ABBREVIATIONS

AI	Artificial Intelligence
AMS	Analog and mixed signal
CAD	Computer aided design
CPU	Central processing unit
DUT	Device under test
GPU	Graphics processing unit
IC	Integrated circuit
KGD	Known good die
ML	Machine Learning
OPC	Optical proximity correction
SEM	Scanning electron microscope
SVM	Support vector machine
VLSI	Very large scale integration

DOI: 10.1201/9781003431138-14

14.1 BACKGROUND

For both health monitoring systems and clinical treatment, it is very important to develop new biomedical devices and circuits that can be carried around or put inside the body. This will help lower the cost of healthcare without sacrificing quality. Therefore, the integrated circuit (IC) industry will have to investigate and develop solutions to decrease design complexity due to increased process variability and lower chip production turnaround time. The traditional methods used are laborious, time-consuming and resource-intensive. However, Artificial Intelligence (AI) unique learning algorithms enable intriguing, automated ways for addressing complicated and data-demanding tasks in VLSI design and testing. Using AI and Machine Learning (ML) techniques in VLSI design and implementation saves the time and energy needed to analyze and process data at various abstraction levels. It increases IC yield and decreases production turnaround time. This chapter covers previous AI/ML automated Very Large-Scale Integration (VLSI) design and production methodologies available in the literature and addresses potential AI/ML applications at multiple abstraction levels to change VLSI design with high-speed, intelligent and efficient implementation.

14.2 INTRODUCTION

As a subfield of applied computer science, VLSI Computer Aided Design (CAD) has always been at the technical vanguard in merging cutting-edge algorithms into software tools and techniques used by electronics engineers to weave the digital fiber of our world, especially in biomedical applications that require VLSI circuits that require less space, are compact and faster [1–4]. This chapter outlines how VLSI CAD has been at the forefront of using ML technology to automate chip design, verification and implementation [5–9]. Machine learning and VLSI CAD may have benefited from their similarities. Moore's law has made billions of transistors commonplace and almost expected. Second, it's an orderly way to manage complexity. Multilayer networks power machine learning inference and generalization. From the transistor's raw data to the chip's processing and computing model, VLSI CAD manages complexity via a well-defined abstraction hierarchy. Third, both domains emphasize computational efficiency, whether to speed up VLSI CAD or to find patterns in time series [10]. Furthermore, VLSI CAD has put a lot of effort into automating optimization and synthesis, which is a trend in the design of neural networks for machine learning.

Expertise in VLSI CAD is crucial in chip design, particularly when dealing with massive volumes of data and designing the processors that initiated the Big Data era. This chapter describes how machine learning has infiltrated semiconductor design [11]. From lithography and physical design to logic and system design and from circuit performance evaluation to yield prediction, VLSI CAD researchers have applied state-of-the-art supervised and unsupervised learning methodologies to pressing CAD issues such as hotspot identification, design-space exploration, effective test generation and post-silicon measurement minimization [12, 13].

Machine learning in VLSI CAD will improve CAD models and chip designs from CAD flows and methodologies. This chapter will show how the osmosis between cognitive structures, methods and hardware designs and technologies will work when cognitive systems and edge intelligence are used in the semiconductor industry.

Automation reduces delays, costs and errors. Automation in VLSI CAD has achieved these goals and created a feedback loop in which computers make other computers that are more powerful. Positive feedback is Moore's law's unseen hand. As we shift from the computer age to the cognitive age, we should recall the success of VLSI CAD and seek the invisible hand that future cognitive systems may create more important cognitive systems. The following structure has been implemented for the chapter's organization: In Section 14.3, we will discuss how machine learning may be used in the lithography process. In Section 14.4, the methodologies of machine learning that were pursued to improve the yield and reliability of IC production are discussed. The applications of machine learning to the design of analogue circuits are discussed in Section 14.5. Finally, the conclusion is in Section 14.6.

14.3 LITHOGRAPHIC AND PHYSICAL DESIGN VIA THE LENS OF MACHINE LEARNING

A technique known as computational lithography may be found buried deep inside the workflow of every contemporary IC manufacturing line. Computational lithography lies at the crossroads of nanofabrication and machine learning [16]. This method implements a software-driven control loop by using massive-scale high-performance computing and an in-depth understanding of nanometric physics, statistics, signal processing and electron microscopy. Computational lithography software is able to successfully control the writing of multilayer patterns on the surfaces of silicon wafers by having the user describe the forms that should be printed on photomasks [17, 18]. These patterns are then etched and deposited. Without this technology, it would not be possible to manufacture the Graphics Processing Unit (GPU) used for today's deep learning training, nor would it be possible to manufacture the Central Processing Unit (CPU) used for the cloud or in cell phones. This method uses electron microscopic pictures to teach a machine learning application. Despite the intimate linkages between machine learning and computational lithography since model-based Optical Proximity Correction (OPC), most practitioners in both domains have developed their work in parallel without realizing their interdependencies. Computational lithography experts have their own language, methodologies and tools [18–21].

Most machine learning researchers aren't familiar with lithographic patterning, although it's vital for expanding chip processing capability, making deep learning cost-effective and realistic. Most technologists are familiar with Moore's law [22], which predicts a rise in the number of transistors on electronic components over time. This section explains how lithographic patterning benefited Moore's law and the pricing of AI and ML. To use machine learning to improve patterning technology, you need to know what the main steps of a patterning process are.

This understanding must be attained before one can learn how to improve patterning technology. Figure 14.1 shows the stages of the patterning process done from the layout stage to the etching stage [23], and Figure 14.2 highlights the compact process machine learning model utilized for optimization. The machine learning problem is stated as: To train through experience E with regard to a certain category of tasks T and efficiency measure P, if its efficiency in tasks in T, as assessed by P, increases with experience E. T stands for the task of figuring out the pattern that was sent to the substrate through a patterning process. E is the testing patterns (input, output) training dataset pairings containing mask layout polygonal inputs and Scanning Electron Microscope (SEM) image output. Performance P is the degree to which the measured and modeled edges of the patterned area match up.

After identifying layout data L, infer the silicon wafer design. The mapping procedure starts by traveling from L to R. When building compact

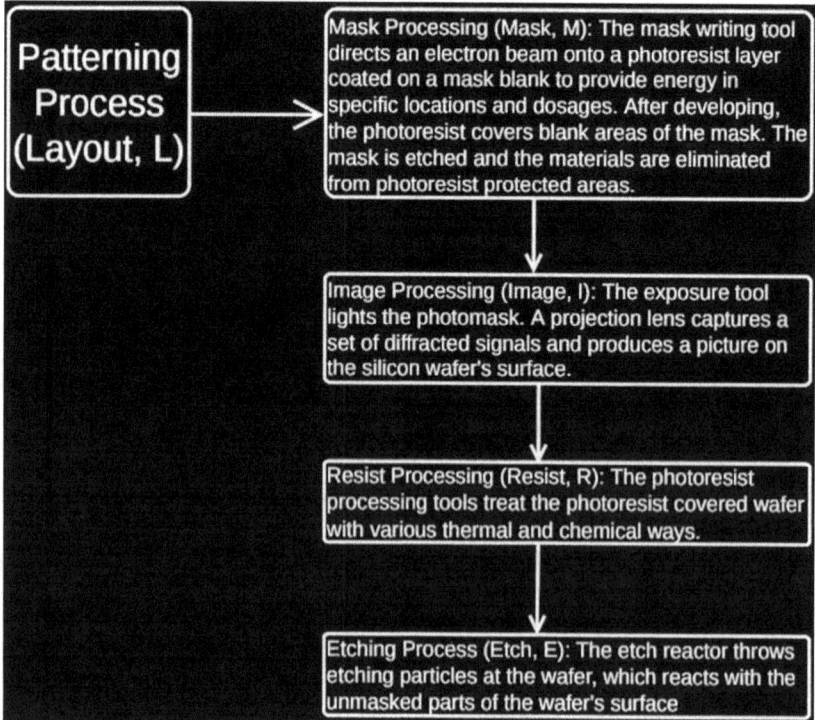

Figure 14.1 Patterning process done from layout stage to the etching stage [23].

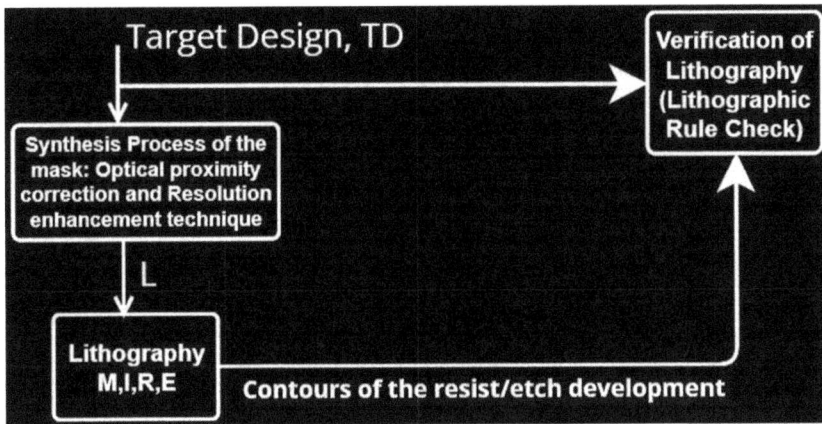

Figure 14.2 Compact process machine learning model utilized for optimization.

process models, lithography teams traditionally prioritize modeling the photoresist pattern. Even though the distribution of the etch contour E is the most important result of lithography, mapping from R to E has been done separately, using rules-based correction/etch process adjustments, or even sometimes a supplemental staged correction with a model that maps directly from the photoresist contour to the etch contour [22].

A suitable coordinate mapping connection is needed to infer the position of the observed contour R in the layout L's coordinate space. Position, scale, rotation and other transform variables must be included. Most test designs allow easy determination of these variables' values. Using symmetric testing and lithography reduces the probability of a placement error. An accurate mapping of the SEM picture to design coordinates is easier if the test pattern has a recognizable pitch, which is common for one-dimensional structures. One-dimensional structures have one dimension. On the other hand, these parameters may be too restrictive for making sure that training data is representative of test situations, which can lead to overfitting [23].

When it comes to the production of integrated circuits, there are often certain combinations of geometries on the input layout L that are of fundamental importance in terms of performance, owing to the frequency with which they arise, and the functional role that they play in the device. One of the most distinguishing features of a certain lithography method, for instance, can be the distance between lines that are next to one another. In the case of these kinds of structures, it is of the utmost significance to reduce the amount of bias present in the model. It is standard practice to provide a measure of maximum absolute prediction error on a limited number of the so-called anchor gauges in order to aid in decreasing bias on chosen features. This helps to reduce bias in selected features. Table 14.1 shows the machine learning methodologies available in the literature.

Table 14.1 Machine learning methodologies available in the literature for lithographic process

Stage	T	E	P	Cost function	Input representation	Output representation	Model form	Training algorithm	Benefit
M [24]	Estimate the dosage modification to enhance M	Dose estimates that have been pre-corrected	Variance in anticipated pixel values	Root Mean Square (RMS) Error	Binary executable 2D pixel map	Scalar valued (dose adjustment)	The logistic regression formula	Gradient Descent Vs Backpropagation	Amount of speed
M [25]	Estimate L to M	Mask 2D SEM Images	Gap between edge positions that were anticipated and those that were measured	RMS Error	Real Valued 2D pixel map	Vector valued location error	A neural network with a single hidden layer that is parallel and has linear outputs	Gradient Descent Vs Backpropagation	Precision
I [26]	An approximation of the spectrum that is diffracted	Diffraction spectra that have been meticulously simulated	Variation in spectra among anticipated and simulated	RMS Error	Real Valued 2D pixel map	4 Real Valued 2D pixel map	Two perceptron with many layers. Activations of the sigmoid. Straight outputs	Gradient Descent Vs Backpropagation	Amount of speed
R	Estimate I to R	2D SEM Images	Variation in position of the edges among anticipated and simulated	RMS Error	Multiple hand-made feature maps with parameters that can be changed	One scalar	Linear	Gradient Descent Vs Backpropagation	Amount of speed
R [27]	Estimate I to R development rate	Simulation curves of development vs exposure intensity	Difference between estimated and simulated development rates	RMS Error	Exposure Intensity and Resist Depth	Rate of Etch	Linear	Gradient Descent Vs Backpropagation	Amount of speed

R [28]	Estimate I to R	2D SEM Images	Variation in position of the edges among anticipated and simulated	RMS Error	1D Vector (Cutline of ariel Image Intensity	1D vector (Cutline of resist I/dose)	Linear	Gradient Descent Vs Backpropagation	Precision
R [29]	Estimate I to R	2D SEM Images	Variation in position of the edges among anticipated and simulated	RMS Error	Real Valued 2D pixel map	One scalar	Linear	Gradient Descent Vs Backpropagation	Precision
R [30]	Estimate L to R	3D simulations of resist	Variation in the resist height among anticipated and simulated	RMS Error	Radial Pattern Density, Convolutions of Bessel functions	One scalar	Multilayer Perceptron, Activation of Sigmoid	Gradient Descent Vs Backpropagation	Amount of speed
R [30]	Estimate R to E	Measurement of etch bias	Variation in the resist height among anticipated and simulated	RMS Error	Radial Pattern Density, Convolutions of Bessel functions	One scalar	Multilayer Perceptron, Activation of Sigmoid	Gradient Descent Vs Backpropagation	Precision

14.4 MACHINE LEARNING APPROACHES TO IMPROVE THE YIELD AND THE RELIABILITY OF IC MANUFACTURING

The production procedures for semiconductors are highly automated and make extensive use of the data that is available. As a result of the inherent unpredictability of nanoscale fabrication as well as its ever-increasing complexity, a variety of data mining and machine learning strategies have been suggested as potential ways to enhance various stages of the manufacturing process [31–34]. In this section, we will look at how machine learning may be used to forecast and improve the yield and reliability of the IC manufacture. To be more explicit, we want to be able to forecast the outcomes of final device testing using data from earlier stages.

14.4.1 ML for Wafer Level Coherence

Unwanted process variations have become an increasingly difficult problem for semiconductor makers to solve as the complexity of current ICs continues to rise while the feature sizes drop significantly. These variances often cause marginalities or even failures, which has an effect on both the quality and production of the product. As a result, having an awareness of, maintaining a monitoring system for, and taking steps to reduce the impact of these variances is essential for assuring the manufacturing of contemporary semiconductor devices. After fabrication, a number of different kinds of tests are carried out in order to get an understanding of how the results of the process modifications impact the functionality and performance of each created device [35, 36].

By studying the fluctuation of wafer-level data, we can detect most failed devices. Every measurement is matched to established specification limitations. This compares devices to decide if they pass or fail (Device Under Test (DUT)). Wafer-level correlation models may enhance these tactics, increasing testing accuracy and reducing test time. We can do this by using numerous correlations. Spatial, temporal, or both correlations may exist between die on the same wafer. Correlations may include e-tests or spec tests. Statistical methods leverage such relationships.

These studies sought to reduce the number of specification tests [37, 38], optimize the test flow at the wafer level [39], and develop machine learning models to identify classification boundaries separating passing and failing populations of devices in a multidimensional space of low-cost measurements [42, 43]. All these studies employ wafer-level testing correlations.

Spatial correlation links a test measurement's position on the wafer to its surroundings. Similar manufacturing processes provide nearby semiconductor areas with similar physical properties. Wafers with similar process characteristics have different temporal work. Manufactured lots are wafers sliced from the same silicon ingot. Wafers within a lot have high temporal

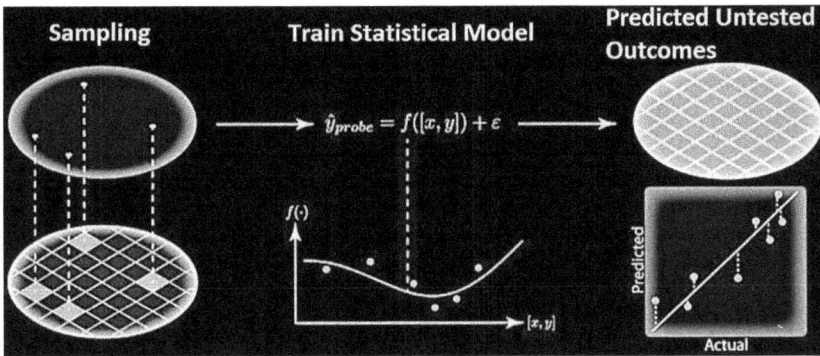

Figure 14.3 Spatial interpolation approach where the statistical model has been trained using sampled wafer data [42].

relationships, but not between lots. Using wafer-level spatial correlations, we can predict unobserved die measurements, allowing us to measure a sparse subset of die. Sample rate affects inaccuracy and time (cost). Figure 14.3 shows spatial interpolation, where a statistical model trained on sampled wafer data predicts the remainder. Any prediction has an error, given as a departure from a 45-degree diagonal [43].

14.4.2 ML for Improving IC Yield

The six high-level IC memory manufacturing procedures are presented in Figure 14.4. In flash memory chip production, wafers are made in wafer fab facilities and then electrically tested. Wafers and dies are marked based on test findings. SME1 and SME2 are the major fabrication tests. These are the electrical experiments at two temperatures. To save money, die that fail SME1 are not tested in SME2. Fabs mark wafers with SME1 and SME2 failed dies. Wafers and data are sent to an assembly and test facility. This facility may "cherry select" wafers based on the fab's test results. A Known Good Die (KGD) test is conducted. Die wafers from various levels undergo distinct KGD methods. Cherry-picked "prime" wafer dies undergo a stringent KGD test and are packed into high-end goods. Packaging follows. Wafers are diced after preparation and processing. Then, dies and passive components are wire-bonded to the substrate. Die stacking is important. The device is then encased [44]. After packing, the final memory test certifies the product's real-world operation. The manufacturing process of the flash memory chip is shown in Figure 14.4. A memory test evaluates each die inside a package, even if they are packed. Memory tests pass or fail each die. All dies chosen for packing have passed thorough electrical testing; however, some fail the final memory test following packaging. There are "really" defective or low-performance dies that were deemed excellent or high-performance by previous tests, and, given the limits of the present

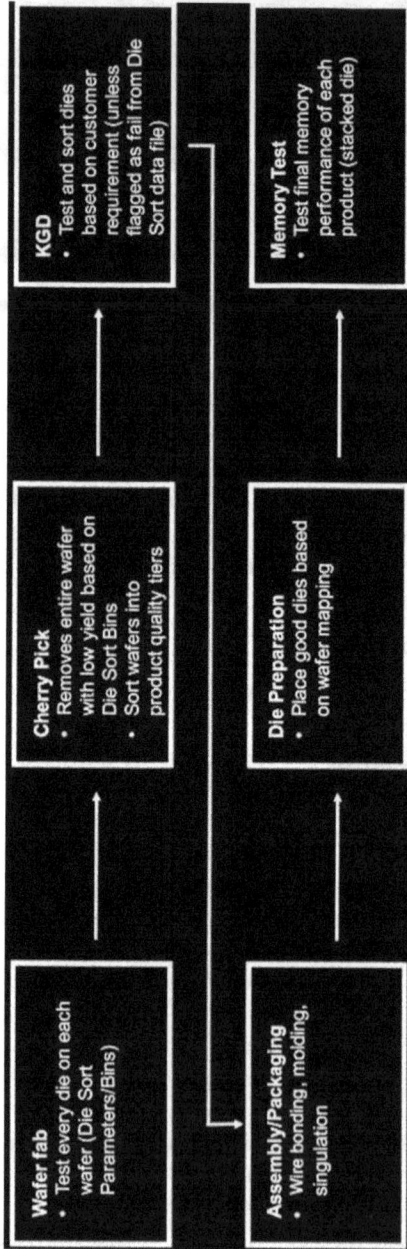

Figure 14.4 The manufacturing process of the flash memory chip [44].

test decision procedure, they can only be found by the final memory test. If only one of the dies inside the package crashes, the entire package fails. The corporation downgrades "failed" bundles into low-end, less profitable ones. Since the quantity of shipments is fixed, the corporation wants high-end items to increase profit. A single failed die may downgrade a whole package, wasting excellent (high-performance) dies [44].

Figure 14.5 depicts the above-mentioned machine learning-based classifier. Figure 14.5 displays an electrically tested wafer die. Based on these measurements, some dies are recognized as malfunctioning (Figure 14.5), while others are sent packing after passing SME1 and SME2 electrical testing. Packing implies all dies operate smoothly. Some unsuccessful deaths (Figure 14.5) are poor, and the final memory test may detect them. If we can build a classifier that can predict the final memory test based on fab die electrical test data, more good dies (Figure 14.5) will be stacked for high-end items.

14.4.3 ML for Characterization of Process Variation

It becomes more difficult to control process variations in nanoscale technologies when integrated circuits are scaled towards finer feature sizes. The ever-increasing variability of the manufacturing process results in the inevitable and considerable introduction of uncertainty into the functioning of the circuit. So, modeling and analyzing these differences to make sure they can be made and improve parametric yields has been made a top priority in the design of integrated circuits today [45, 46]. Statistical analysis and optimization of integrated circuits, such as design centering, statistical timing analysis [47, 48], as well as post-silicon tuning [48–51], have been put forward as ways to achieve the above-mentioned goal. These techniques try to predict and, as a result, reduce variations in circuit-level performance. This is done to make a design that is strong and has a high parametric yield. The accuracy of the variation models such as distribution and correlation, which give vital information about manufacturing uncertainties, is a big part of how well these methods work. However, it is not easy to get the variation model right. Silicon wafers and chips should be carefully tested as well as characterized using a variety of test structures, such as I-V structures as well as ring oscillators, that are placed in the scribe lines of the wafer or on the product chips [51–56]. The traditional way of describing silicon has three big problems:

1. Significant area overhead: Most modern microprocessor chips have hundreds of on chip ring oscillators to measure and track parameter changes, which consumes a significant amount of silicon area [53].
2. Long testing time: Physically measuring all test structures across a small number of input/output ports takes a long time. In nanoscale

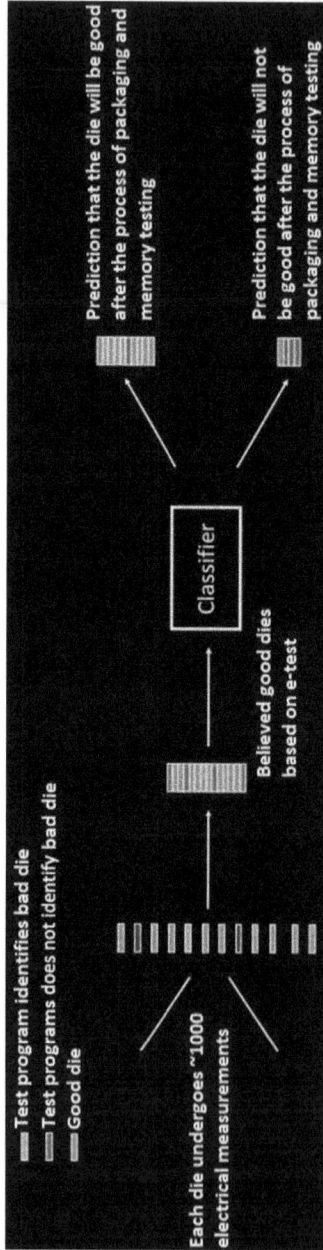

Figure 14.5 Machine learning based classifier for classifying wafers [44].

technologies, testing integrated circuits has added a big chunk to the total cost of making them [57].

3. Testing isn't very reliable: Testing an integrated circuit may even hurt the wafer or chip being tested. For example, mechanical stress from a wafer probe test could damage the wafer in a way that can't be fixed [54].

When these difficulties combine, silicon characterization costs rise because additional test structures are needed to contain tiny devices' spatial shifts. Silicon characterization has been researched before, but a cheaper, more efficient technique is needed now.

14.4.4 ML for Aging Assessment

Bias temperature instability has been one of the main reasons that digital circuits can fail or break down as they age. So, the circuitry has a pessimistic guard band to make sure they are resilient. Integrated circuits made at nanoscale technology nodes can't rely on design time solutions as well as guard bands to keep them safe. This is because the making process, the amount of work and the working conditions vary a lot, which makes developing solutions inefficient and not useful [58, 59]. Because of this, there is a need for runtime solutions that are based on monitoring and changing in real time. Chipmakers utilize voltage or frequency scaling, body biasing and thermal management to cope with slowdowns caused by age, excessive temperature, current surges and so forth. Fixed adaptation policies Lookup tables, booting ROMs, etc., are the hard code system choices required. Adaptation techniques used today are more reactive than predictive, and there's no way to teach certain processes to change as the chip's behavior changes. Figure 14.6 displays SVM modeling aging based on signal probabilities. This approach measures online workload-induced aging-stress as a runtime software thread. Only a limited number of flip-flops in a design must be checked during runtime. This cuts down on the hardware cost of watching and makes it easier for the computer to do its job [59].

14.5 MACHINE LEARNING APPROACHES FOR ANALOG DESIGN

As technology improves, it's getting tougher to develop and construct high-performance analog and mixed-signal circuits. Flexible post-silicon adjustment might help scale AMS circuits continuously. This solves the AMS circuit difficulties. Post-silicon tweaking creates additional design issues. [60–62]. Each analog mixed signal circuit is a vast, sophisticated system that may vary over time. Validation should be done before fixing on silicon. A tunable mixed signal circuit must contain control knobs (switches, adjustable

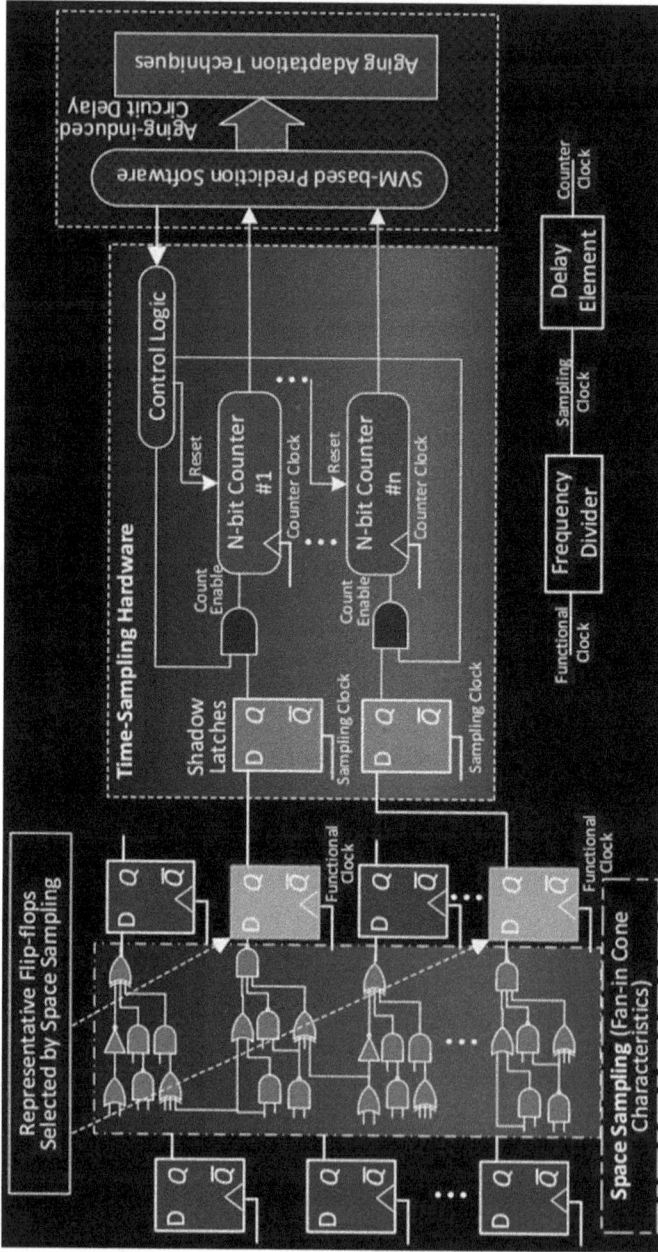

Figure 14.6 Support vector machine model that can predict aging based on signal probabilities [59].

bias voltage or current, etc.) to modify its operation once it has been built. Some chips feature self-healing sensors and control blocks. As a result, the complexity and cost of modeling these circuits for pre-silicon validation increase. This cost problem is particularly critical for complex mixed-signal circuits, like phase-locked loops and high-speed input/output connections, where a single transistor-level simulation might take days or weeks to complete. Validating a design is costly.

We should carry out a number of simulations of process and environmental variables. First, we must test the circuit's performance using on-chip sensors or external equipment. We may configure all the control knobs based on the measurements.

To fulfill these aims, a tuning strategy must relate knob settings to quality. In addition to learning a tuning strategy for all process and environmental circumstances, we must gather plenty of measurement data [63–66]. The tuning policy must be re-calibrated to account for process changes. More measurements are needed. Silicon data might be costly or hard to get since measuring it takes so long [66–68] use Bayesian Model Fusion to address difficulties. Most conventional approaches for verifying and optimizing AMS only employ data acquired in a single step. BMF uses early data to verify and optimize AMS circuits later. So, late-stage data reduction is possible.

14.6 CONCLUSION

Creating new portable and/or surgically implanted biomedical devices and circuits is very important if we want to lower the cost of health care without sacrificing quality. With all of these implantable circuits for different medical uses, billions of US dollars might be saved by updating the current health care infrastructure. The one-of-a-kind learning algorithms that AI employs make possible fascinating automated approaches to the difficult and data-intensive activities that are involved in VLSI development and testing. It is possible to reduce the amount of time and effort needed to analyze and process data at various abstraction levels by using AI and ML approaches in the design and implementation of nanoscale VLSI circuits specifically for biomedical circuits. This improves IC yield while reducing the amount of time needed for manufacturing turnaround. In this chapter we addressed potential AI/ML applications at numerous abstraction levels to change VLSI design with high-speed, smart and efficient implementation and tried to cover previous AI/ML automated VLSI design and production methodologies that are available in the literature. Our study provides a basic infrastructure that makes it possible to design and optimize next-generation biomedical circuits for many new applications.

REFERENCES

[1] Bajaj, Varun, and G. R. Sinha, eds. *Computer-aided Design and Diagnosis Methods for Biomedical Applications*. CRC Press, Boca Raton, Florida, 2021.

[2] Sowmya, Nagavarapu, Shasanka Sekhar Rout, and Rajesh Kumar Patjoshi. "Implementation of ultra-low-power electronics for biomedical applications." In *Electronic Devices, Circuits, and Systems for Biomedical Applications*, pp. 153–176. Academic Press, United States, 2021.

[3] Gupta, Deepika. "Low-voltage analog integrated circuit design." In *Nanoscale VLSI*, pp. 3–22. Springer, Singapore, 2020.

[4] Hung, Chung-Chih, and Shih-Hsing Wang. "Low-power and low-voltage VLSI circuit design techniques for biomedical applications." In *Ultra-Low-Voltage Frequency Synthesizer and Successive-Approximation Analog-to-Digital Converter for Biomedical Applications*, pp. 23–54. Springer, Cham, 2022.

[5] Beerel, Peter A., and Massoud Pedram. "Opportunities for machine learning in electronic design automation." In *2018 IEEE International Symposium on Circuits and Systems (ISCAS)*, pp. 1–5. Florence, Italy , IEEE, 2018.

[6] Joshi, Siddharth, Chul Kim, Sohmyung Ha, and Gert Cauwenberghs. "From algorithms to devices: Enabling machine learning through ultra-low-power VLSI mixed-signal array processing." In *2017 IEEE Custom Integrated Circuits Conference (CICC)*, pp. 1–9. IEEE, 2017.

[7] Boning, Duane S., Ibrahim Abe M. Elfadel, and Xin Li. "A preliminary taxonomy for machine learning in VLSI CAD." In *Machine Learning in VLSI Computer-Aided Design*, pp. 1–16. Springer, Cham, 2019.

[8] Yao, Enyi, and Arindam Basu. "VLSI extreme learning machine: A design space exploration." *IEEE Transactions on Very Large Scale Integration (VLSI) Systems* 25, no. 1 (2016): 60–74.

[9] Mitchell, Tom M., Sridbar Mabadevan, and Louis I. Steinberg. "LEAP: A learning apprentice for VLSI design." In *Machine Learning*, pp. 271–289. Morgan Kaufmann, Elsevier, Netherlands, 1990.

[10] Yu, Bei, David Z. Pan, Tetsuaki Matsunawa, and Xuan Zeng. "Machine learning and pattern matching in physical design." In *The 20th Asia and South Pacific Design Automation Conference*, pp. 286–293. IEEE, 2015.

[11] Batra, Gaurav, Zach Jacobson, Siddarth Madhav, Andrea Queirolo, and Nick Santhanam. "Artificial-intelligence hardware: New opportunities for semiconductor companies." McKinsey Co. December (2018).

[12] Ziegler, Matthew M., Ramon Bertran, Alper Buyuktosunoglu, and Pradip Bose. "Machine learning techniques for taming the complexity of modern hardware design." *IBM Journal of Research and Development* 61, no. 4/5 (2017): 13–1.

[13] Cho, Chang-Burm, James Poe, Tao Li, and Jingling Yuan. "Accurate, scalable and informative design space exploration for large and sophisticated multi-core oriented architectures." In *2009 IEEE International Symposium on Modeling, Analysis & Simulation of Computer and Telecommunication Systems*, pp. 1–10. IEEE, 2009.

[14] Swaminathan, Karthik, Nandhini Chandramoorthy, Chen-Yong Cher, Ramon Bertran, Alper Buyuktosunoglu, and Pradip Bose. "Bravo: Balanced reliability-aware voltage optimization." In *2017 IEEE International Symposium on High Performance Computer Architecture (HPCA)*, pp. 97–108. IEEE, 2017.

[15] Shiely, J. P. "Machine learning for compact lithographic process models." In *Machine Learning in VLSI Computer-Aided Design*, pp. 19–68. Springer, Cham, 2019.

[16] Adam, Kostas, Shashidhara Ganjugunte, Clement Moyroud, Kostya Shchehlik, Michael Lam, Andrew Burbine, Germain Fenger, and Yuri Granik. "Using machine learning in the physical modeling of lithographic processes." In *Design-Process- Technology Co-optimization for Manufacturability XIII*, vol. 10962, pp. 86–93. SPIE, 2019.

[17] Cao, Yu, Ya Luo, Yen-Wen Lu, C. H. E. N. Been-Der, Rafael C. Howell, Yi Zou, Jing Su, and S. U. N. Dezheng. "Methods for training machine learning model for computation lithography." U.S. Patent Application 16/970,648, filed December 3, 2020.

[18] Hurley, Paul, and Krzysztof Kryszczuk. "Replacing design rules in the VLSI design cycle." In *Design for Manufacturability through Design-Process Integration VI*, vol. 8327, pp. 100–105. SPIE, 2012.

[19] Shin, Youngsoo. "Computational lithography using machine learning models." *IPSJ Transactions on System LSI Design Methodology* 14 (2021): 2–10.

[20] Shim, Seongbo, Suhyeong Choi, and Youngsoo Shin. "Machine learning for mask synthesis." In *Machine Learning in VLSI Computer-Aided Design*, pp. 69–93. Springer, Cham, 2019.

[21] Moore, Gordon E. "Cramming more components onto integrated circuits." (1965): 114–117.

[22] Rieger, Michael L. "Communication theory in optical lithography." *Journal of Micro/Nanolithography, MEMS, and MOEMS* 11, no. 1 (2012): 013003.

[23] Frye, Robert C., Edward A. Rietman, and Kevin D. Cummings. "Neural network proximity effect corrections for electron beam lithography." In *1990 IEEE International Conference on Systems, Man, and Cybernetics Conference Proceedings*, pp. 704–706. IEEE, 1990.

[24] Nakayamada, Noriaki, Rieko Nishimura, Satoru Miura, Haruyuki Nomura, and Takashi Kamikubo. "Electron beam lithographic modeling assisted by artificial intelligence technology." In *Photomask Japan 2017: XXIV Symposium on Photomask and Next-Generation Lithography Mask Technology*, vol. 10454, p. 104540B. International Society for Optics and Photonics, 2017.

[25] Agudelo, Viviana, Tim Fühner, Andreas Erdmann, and Peter Evanschitzky. "Application of artificial neural networks to compact mask models in optical lithography simulation." *Journal of Micro/Nanolithography, MEMS, and MOEMS* 13, no. 1 (2013): 011002.

[26] Sturtevant, John, and Luigi Capodieci. "Design for Manufacturing and Design Process Technology Co-Optimization." In *Microlithography*, pp. 293–326. CRC Press, Boca Raton, Florida, 2020.

[27] Zach, Franz X. "Neural-network-based approach to resist modeling and opc." In *Optical Microlithography XVII*, vol. 5377, pp. 670–679. SPIE, 2004.

[28] Watanabe, Yuki, Taiki Kimura, Tetsuaki Matsunawa, and Shigeki Nojima. "Accurate lithography simulation model based on convolutional neural networks." In *Optical Microlithography XXX*, vol. 10147, p. 101470K. International Society for Optics and Photonics, 2017.

[29] S. Shim et al., Machine learning-based resist 3D model. *Proc. SPIE* 10147 (2017).

[30] Shim, Seongbo, and Youngsoo Shin. "Etch proximity correction through machine-learning-driven etch bias model." In *Advanced Etch Technology for Nanopatterning V*, vol. 9782, p. 978200. International Society for Optics and Photonics, 2016.

[31] Hasani, Hamid, Seyed Mohammad Jafar Jalali, Danial Rezaei, and Mohsen Maleki. "A data mining framework for classification of organisational performance based on rough set theory." *Asian Journal of Management Science and Applications* 3, no. 2 (2018): 156–180.

[32] Park, In-Beom, Jaeseok Huh, Joongkyun Kim, and Jonghun Park. "A reinforcement learning approach to robust scheduling of semiconductor manufacturing facilities." *IEEE Transactions on Automation Science and Engineering* 17, no. 3 (2019): 1420–1431.

[33] Mizuno, Shigeru, and Norman Bodek. *Management for Quality Improvement: The Seven New QC Tools*. Productivity Press, New York 2020.

[34] Weiss, Sholom M., Amit Dhurandhar, and Robert J. Baseman. "Improving quality control by early prediction of manufacturing outcomes." In *Proceedings of the 19th ACM SIGKDD International Conference on Knowledge Discovery and Data Mining*, pp. 1258–1266. 2013.

[35] Chen, Hongge. "Novel machine learning approaches for modeling variations in semiconductor manufacturing." PhD diss., Massachusetts Institute of Technology, 2017.

[36] Geurkov, Vadim, and Lev Kirischian. "A Unified Method of Designing Signature Analyzers for Digital and Mixed-Signal Circuits Testing." In *2020 IEEE International Test Conference (ITC)*, pp. 1–5. IEEE, 2020.

[37] Brockman, Jay B., and Stephen W. Director. "Predictive subset testing: Optimizing IC parametric performance testing for quality, cost, and yield." *IEEE Transactions on Semiconductor Manufacturing* 2, no. 3 (1989): 104–113.

[38] Ahmadi, Ali, Amit Nahar, Bob Orr, Michael Past, and Yiorgos Makris. "Wafer-level process variation-driven probe-test flow selection for test cost reduction in analog/RF ICs." In *2016 IEEE 34th VLSI Test Symposium (VTS)*, pp. 1–6. IEEE, 2016.

[39] Niranjan, V. A., Deepika Neethirajan, Constantinos Xanthopoulos, E. De La Rosa, C. Alleyne, S. Mier, and Yiorgos Makris. "Trim Time Reduction in Analog/RF ICs Based on Inter-Trim Correlation." In *2021 IEEE 39th VLSI Test Symposium (VTS)*, pp. 1–7. IEEE, 2021.

[40] Voorakaranam, Ram, Selim Sermet Akbay, Soumendu Bhattacharya, Sasikumar Cherubal, and Abhijit Chatterjee. "Signature testing of analog and RF circuits: Algorithms and methodology." *IEEE Transactions on Circuits and Systems I: Regular Papers* 54, no. 5 (2007): 1018–1031.

[41] Stratigopoulos, Haralampos-G., and Yiorgos Makris. "Error moderation in low-cost machine-learning-based analog/RF testing." *IEEE Transactions on Computer-Aided Design of Integrated Circuits and Systems* 27, no. 2 (2008): 339–351.

[42] Stratigopoulos, Haralampos-G., Petros Drineas, Mustapha Slamani, and Yiorgos Makris. "RF specification test compaction using learning machines." *IEEE Transactions on Very Large Scale Integration (VLSI) Systems* 18, no. 6 (2009): 998–1002.

[43] Jiang, Dan, Weihua Lin, and Nagarajan Raghavan. "A novel framework for semiconductor manufacturing final test yield classification using machine learning techniques." *IEEE Access* 8 (2020): 197885–197895.

[44] Najafi-Haghi, Zahra Paria, Marzieh Hashemipour-Nazari, and Hans-Joachim Wunderlich. "Variation-aware defect charac- terization at cell level." In *2020 IEEE European Test Symposium (ETS)*, pp. 1–6. IEEE, 2020.

[45] Nayak, Peshal. "A Study of Technology Roadmap for Application-Specific Integrated Circuit." PhD diss., Rice University, 2021.

[46] Chang, Hongliang, and Sachin S. Sapatnekar. "Statistical timing analysis under spatial correlations." *IEEE Transactions on Computer-Aided Design of Integrated Circuits and Systems* 24, no. 9 (2005): 1467–1482.

[47] Visweswariah, Chandramouli, Kaushik Ravindran, Kerim Kalafala, Steven G. Walker, Sambasivan Narayan, Daniel K. Beece, Jeff Piaget, Natesan Venkateswaran, and Jeffrey G. Hemmett. "First-order incremental block-based statistical timing analysis." *IEEE Transactions on Computer-Aided Design of Integrated Circuits and Systems* 25, no. 10 (2006): 2170–2180.

[48] Zhan, Yaping, Andrzej J. Strojwas, Xin Li, Lawrence T. Pileggi, David Newmark, and Mahesh Sharma. "Correlation-aware statistical timing analysis with non-Gaussian delay distributions." In *Proceedings of the 42nd Annual Design Automation Conference*, pp. 77–82. 2005.

[49] Heloue, Khaled R., and Farid N. Najm. "Statistical timing analysis with two-sided constraints." In *ICCAD-2005. IEEE/ACM International Conference on Computer-Aided Design, 2005*, pp. 829–836. IEEE, 2005.

[50] Mani, Murari, Ashish K. Sing, and Michael Orshansky. "Joint design-time and post-silicon minimization of parametric yield loss using adjustable robust opti-mization." In *Proceedings of the 2006 IEEE/ACM international conference on Computer- aided design*, pp. 19–26. 2006.

[51] Ketchen, Mark, M. Bhushan, and D. Pearson. "High speed test structures for in-line process monitoring and model calibration [CMOS applications]." In *Proceedings of the 2005 International Conference on Microelectronic Test Structures, 2005. ICMTS 2005*, pp. 33–38. IEEE, 2005.

[52] Bhushan, Manjul, Anne Gattiker, Mark B. Ketchen, and Koushik K. Das. "Ring oscillators for CMOS process tuning and variability control." *IEEE Transactions on Semiconductor Manufacturing* 19, no. 1 (2006): 10–18.

[53] Mann, William R., Frederick L. Taber, Philip W. Seitzer, and Jerry J. Broz. "The leading edge of production wafer probe test technology." In *2004 International Conference on Test*, pp. 1168–1195. IEEE, 2004.

[54] Koushanfar, Farinaz, Petros Boufounos, and Davood Shamsi. "Post-silicon timing characterization by compressed sensing." In *2008 IEEE/ACM International Conference on Computer-Aided Design*, pp. 185–189. IEEE, 2008.

[55] Reda, Sherief, and Sani R. Nassif. "Analyzing the impact of process varia-tions on parametric measurements: Novel models and applications." In *2009 Design, Automation & Test in Europe Conference & Exhibition*, pp. 375–380. IEEE, 2009.

[56] Bushnell, Michael, and Vishwani Agrawal. *Essentials of Electronic Testing for Digital, Memory and Mixed-Signal VLSI Circuits*, vol. 17. Springer Science & Business Media, 2004.

[57] Fojtik, Matthew, David Fick, Yejoong Kim, Nathaniel Pinckney, David Harris, David Blaauw, and Dennis Sylvester. "Bub- ble Razor: An architecture-inde-pendent approach to timing-error detection and correction." In *2012 IEEE International Solid-State Circuits Conference*, pp. 488–490. IEEE, 2012.

[58] Vijayan, Arunkumar, Krishnendu Chakrabarty, and Mehdi B. Tahoori. "Machine Learning-Based Aging Analysis." In *Machine Learning in VLSI Computer-Aided Design*, pp. 265–289. Springer, Cham, 2019.

[59] Tang, Adrian, Frank Hsiao, David Murphy, I-Ning Ku, Jenny Liu, Sandeep D'Souza, Ning-Yi Wang et al. "A low-overhead self-healing embedded system for ensuring high yield and long-term sustainability of 60GHz 4Gb/s radio-on-a-chip." In *2012 IEEE International Solid-State Circuits Conference*, pp. 316–318. IEEE, 2012.

[60] Bowers, Steven M., Kaushik Sengupta, Kaushik Dasgupta, and Ali Hajimiri. "A fully-integrated self-healing power amplifier." In *2012 IEEE Radio Frequency Integrated Circuits Symposium*, pp. 221–224. IEEE, 2012.

[61] Plouchart, Jean-Olivier, Mark A. Ferriss, Arun S. Natarajan, Alberto Valdes-Garcia, Bodhisatwa Sadhu, Alexander Rylyakov, Benjamin D. Parker et al. "A 23.5 GHz PLL with an adaptively biased VCO in 32 nm SOI-CMOS." *IEEE Transactions on Circuits and Systems I: Regular Papers* 60, no. 8 (2013): 2009–2017.

[62] Kupp, Nathan, He Huang, Petros Drineas, and Yiorgos Makris. "Post-production performance calibration in analog/RF devices." In *2010 IEEE International Test Conference*, pp. 1–10. IEEE, 2010.

[63] Han, Donghoon, Byung Sung Kim, and Abhijit Chatterjee. "DSP-driven self-tuning of RF circuits for process-induced performance variability." *IEEE Transactions on Very Large Scale Integration (VLSI) Systems* 18, no. 2 (2009): 305–314.

[64] Roy, Soham, Spencer K. Millican, and Vishwani D. Agrawal. "Special session–machine learning in test: A survey of analog, digital, memory, and rf integrated circuits." In *2021 IEEE 39th VLSI Test Symposium (VTS)*, pp. 1–14. IEEE, 2021.

[65] Tao, Jun, Fa Wang, Paolo Cachecho, Wangyang Zhang, Shupeng Sun, Xin Li, Rouwaida Kanj, Chenjie Gu, and Xuan Zeng. "Large-scale circuit performance modeling by bayesian model fusion." In *Machine Learning in VLSI Computer-Aided Design*, pp. 403–422. Springer, Cham, 2019.

[66] Wang, Mengshuo, Fan Yang, Changhao Yan, Xuan Zeng, and Xiangdong Hu. "Efficient Bayesian yield optimization approach for analog and SRAM circuits." In *2017 54th ACM/EDAC/IEEE Design Automation Conference (DAC)*, pp. 1–6. IEEE, 2017.

[67] Zeng, Wei, Hengliang Zhu, Xuan Zeng, Dian Zhou, Rueywen Liu, and Xin Li. "C-yes: An efficient parametric yield estimation approach for analog and mixed-signal circuits based on multicorner-multiperformance correlations." *IEEE Transactions on Computer-Aided Design of Integrated Circuits and Systems* 36, no. 6 (2016): 899–912.

[68] Wang, Fa, Paolo Cachecho, Wangyang Zhang, Shupeng Sun, Xin Li, Rouwaida Kanj, and Chenjie Gu. "Bayesian model fusion: large-scale performance modeling of analog and mixed-signal circuits by reusing early-stage data." *IEEE Transactions on Computer-Aided Design of Integrated Circuits and Systems* 35, no. 8 (2015): 1255–1268.

Index

For Product Safety Concerns and Information please contact our EU
representative GPSR@taylorandfrancis.com
Taylor & Francis Verlag GmbH, Kaufingerstraße 24, 80331 München, Germany

www.ingramcontent.com/pod-product-compliance
Lightning Source LLC
Chambersburg PA
CBHW070712220326
41598CB00024BA/3120